Lessons Earned

Cancer As A Catalyst

By

Kimball Walker

Kimball Walker books are available
for order through Ingram Press Catalogues

This book is not intended as a substitute for the medical
advice of physicians. The reader should regularly consult a
physician in matters relating to his/her health and particularly
with respect to any symptoms that may require diagnosis or
medical attention. Also, the information in this book is meant
to supplement, not replace proper nutrition and exercise.
The authors and publisher advise readers to take full
responsibility for their safety and know their limits.
Lessons Earned is not about taking any risks beyond your
level of aptitude or comfort.

Kimball Walker
Visit my website at www.higherguidancehealing.com

Printed in the United States of America
First Printing: December 2014
Published by Sojourn Publishing, LLC

ISBN: 978-1-62747-100-8
Ebook ISBN: 978-1-62747-101-5
LCN: Pending

Acknowledgements

2 010 was a year of wonder for me and it began with the amount of help I received from so many people. Cancer may be a big business, but it also brings out the best in people – caregivers, doctors and friends. My immediate family was tremendously supportive even when I went outside the lines, but it was also a daily occurrence for total strangers to help me out. Even today, I can't go back to that time without it bringing tears to my eyes.

I'd like to thank my family: Jeff, John and Ali for giving me a reason to be strong and to change everything. My sisters and especially, my sister Pam who is unendingly giving, talented and who has never not been there for me. Annie and Laurie who put me up and put up with me during and after - thank you. Harry and Carol for 26 years of unending support, but especially, Carol, thank you for all the love and help during my cancer year - you were my pillar.

I don't know how I got to be so fortunate, but my girlfriends are stellar and although I can't mention them all…I have to thank those here in alphabetical order because you're all fabulous….Alayne, for keeping the faith. Jeannie, for your unique and brilliant perspective and all the years of showing up. Julie, for being my biggest influence in the last ten years – yay! Laura, for sharing yourself with me. Lisa, for 25 years of the best kind of friend any girl could ask for. Louise, for being so faithful. Maggie, for being absolutely Maggie. Sharon, for teaching me to soften and your kind, loving support. Valerie, for 28 years and standing in when I couldn't stand. Stef, for almost 40 years of sisterhood. Pam, for being my spiritual guide, giving months of your time and being there during the tough stuff. And my trusted best girlfriend, Meka, who has never left my side since she was two months old.

Sedona captured me the minute I saw my first red rock – I knew I would live here after that. Thank you for taking me in and embracing me, supporting me and being so welcoming – you are my home now. Your mountains fill me up like nothing I've ever known. Sedona brought me to Tom Bird, who brought me to RamaJon and without RamaJon, I never would have written this book.

Thanks Rama.

Contents

Introduction... vii
1. A Miracle 1
2. The Beginning.. 9
3. A No-Brainer 17
4. Creative Recovery.. 19
5. Alkaline Diet... 23
6. Eating with Attitude.................................... 35
7. Leave the Wine Behind............................... 39
8. Pray for Peace 43
9. The Elixir of Life 47
10. Reading Your Body 51
11. A Meditation for Healing.......................... 59
12. Stress on the Body 63
13. Nurturing.. 65
14. Moving... 67
15. Higher Guidance 73
16. A Healthy Point of View........................... 83
17. Getting Quiet.. 85
18. Mirror Meditation 89
19. Manifesting Health.................................... 91
20. Habits 101
21. Zoning Out.. 107
22. Habits Become Character 111

23. Your Story 115
24. Pain Gives Way to Peace 121
25. Are You a Victim? 127
26. Power versus Pity 135
27. Changing my Story 141
28. Stress Memory 145
29. The Body's Reflexes 151
30. Believe It and Become It 155
31. It's Never Finished 165
32. Being Heard 169
33. Losing Self-Consciousness 173
34. What's Focus Got to Do with It? 175
35. Preparing for Power 181
36. Personality 187
37. Goodness 197
38. Viewpoint 205
39. Gratitude 213
40. Journaling 219
41. You Have You 225
42. Living outside the Lines 229
43. Forgiveness 235
44. Lesson Earned 243
45. Faith's the Opposite of Fear 251
46. Sharing Your Truth 259
47. Authenticity 265
48. Creating Your World 269
49. No Such Thing 277
50. Finding Your Tribe 285
51. Risk It 289
52. You Have to Remember You 295
53. Grounded 301
54. A Different Level 307

Introduction

W hen you have been given a diagnosis of cancer, your world becomes focused instantly and you wonder, *What do I have to do to get well?*

You know you'll need doctors, possibly surgery and treatments, time off from work, insurance coverage, and tremendous support. One out of eight women will get breast cancer in their lifetime.[*] In 2013, there were more than 2.8 million with a history of breast cancer in the U.S. and that's just breast cancer. This is something that one way or another will affect us all.

What if you knew that getting cancer would be a good thing? What if the reason you got cancer was to wake up to a better you? What if you knew that in undergoing such an ordeal you were going to get stronger, more spiritual, more loving, and more sure of yourself than you've ever been? What if you ended up being happier than you were before you had it? Would it make it easier for you to get through?

What if getting cancer was all for your own good?

---

[*]   breastcancer.org/symtoms/understand_bc/statistics

If you knew, when you were diagnosed with cancer, that it would be an uplifting, life-changing experience, you could begin the journey without fear and dread. Right? You need to know that all the pain, the despair, and the fear is not necessary, but if and when it comes, it's worth it. You need to know that you can come out on the other side a new person who will be stronger than ever — and filled with new wisdom.

What if getting well had more to do with your attitude than you thought? What I learned during my year of cancer was more about training my mind than anything else. I was shocked to discover that what I was thinking had helped make me sick. I was even more surprised to find that I could control my thoughts and shape my daily experience.

I know that some of our lives might be shorter than others. There isn't any one of us who has gone through this that doesn't have a heightened sense of their mortality. I am not brushing over the fact that cancer will take some of us before we're ready. That's not the point. The point is that when you live your days fully, and with a grateful attitude, you won't think about the future as something that matters more than right now. Today is what matters. There is no guarantee for anybody. When you make each day a masterpiece, you can let go of the tomorrows. Tomorrow isn't here yet and this is freedom. That can change your life more than any other one thing.

Frankly, this book is about a metamorphosis brought on by panic. I admit it: I panicked. My life did a complete U-turn. I started on this journey just trying to change enough so I would get well, and it turned into an exploration of self so deep that there was no turning back. I wouldn't be the same afterwards, but I didn't know that then. I was so tied to myself at the time — the idea of me — that the thought of never being the same would have stopped me in my tracks. I would have refused the lesson.

I didn't know there was more to life than what I was experiencing. I was existing and going through the motions, but not living fully. I'd like to share what I've learned, or more truthfully, what I earned. Because, as I found out, I needed some lessons, and trust me, I finally got them.

The things that I talk about here are what we all already know. Our higher Self has the wisdom of all the ages. It's in there, in your head and your heart. You already own it. I didn't know I had the knowledge until I recognized it all again. There is nothing that you don't already understand — you have just forgotten it. We all need to be reminded sometimes of what's important. I think getting cancer can be that reminder.

The continuous, long-term gratitude I have for what happened to me makes me want to share my experience. Not all of us will be affected the same way, but so much had happened to me that was beneficial - I feel driven to explain what I did and what I learned.

Along the way, I began to treat myself differently, and I'm giving cancer the credit for my good fortune and good feelings. I learned how to nurture myself — to find my authentic self again and to take care of my inner health by finding out what was happening in my body, both physically and emotionally. I found balance and awareness in everything I was doing. I connected to who I truly was and discovered what I was missing in my life.

I'll share a little of my history and what I've learned about health, love, spirituality, and creativity. This book is about looking for and finding the authentic you in and under all the busyness, all the obligations, and all the false faces that you wear. The roles that we play are many. When they hide who you truly are, and, in a lot of cases, make you sick, that's when you need to let them go. Somehow, along the way, we forget who we are and what we know to be true. With some effort, we can find ourselves again.

– 1 –
A Miracle

There are days in your life that you'll never forget — they are the days that shape you and possibly rock the world as you know it. Sometimes you experience events that make you very happy or go through circumstances that have the complete opposite effect. It all comes down to what you do with those days that makes you who you are, and either keeps things coming at you the same way or changes how you go forward forever. I have a story about being rocked — actually more than once.

When I was diagnosed with cancer, I changed almost everything that I'd been doing. I didn't set out to do this. I set out to live through the cancer ordeal and completely recover, but it didn't make sense for me to keep doing what I was doing if it had made me sick. I used cancer as a motivator to get to a new place and become a new me. It wasn't intentional at first, but it became more and more clear that I was changing when my relationships weren't the same and I had difficulty understanding my old ways of thinking. I learned and grew so much that my marriage wasn't the same, my friendships shifted, and I saw my children in a new way.

The biggest thing that happened because of my shift in perspective came when I was faced with the end of my life as I knew it — but not because of cancer. I had recovered from the cancer, only to find more challenges facing me. I had done what I'd set out to do, and living was taking on a new meaning for me. I'd learned how to forgive, to allow, and to let resentments dissolve. This was a crucial aspect of my recovery. Holding on to the experiences that had hurt me was a big part of why I had gotten sick in the first place, and I learned beyond a doubt that forgiveness was where I had healed.

The belief in forgiveness is what made it possible to move through an event that would have most likely sent me down the road to illness again. I wasn't about to go down that road if I didn't have to. All that I had worked for the two years prior was at stake. If I didn't know how to forgive, basically, it had all been for nothing.

The interesting part of what happened was that I didn't intend to forgive at that time, but I think I'd been on the path long enough that I'd put the practice in place. Forgiving was familiar to me now, and the repercussions were obvious. The practice combined with the knowledge of what forgiveness was worth helped me through a very dark time.

The reason I mention this in the beginning of my story is to demonstrate what I learned with the experience of cancer and how much it helped me get through the next troubled time. The overall benefit of cancer for me was beyond compare. If you knew prior to the start of any journey that there'd be an amazingly positive result, you'd take that first step with an inner strength and faith that all would be alright. Actually, any big, potentially scary event can be looked at through the same kind of eyes that I've seen my year with cancer through. All difficult experiences can be beneficial – it's all about how you view it. Although I didn't know at the time, I would need all that I had learned and then some for the next step on my path.

On the morning of February 2, 2013, three years to the day that I was diagnosed with stage 4 breast cancer, I was served with foreclosure papers. What I thought my future would hold was wiped away in the length of time it took to open a certified letter. Through a series of events, a lot of them totally unknown to me, the bank was taking my house and my business with it. I was now faced with debt beyond what I thought possible, and from my vantage point, it all seemed to be my husband's fault. While I was in the dark about what was going on, he was not.

At the time this happened, we had already decided to get a divorce and had our business and home on the market. The foreclosure notices meant that we would get nothing out of the property and I would be left in debt instead of having money to go forward with my life. It was devastating and I was furious and resentful.

Three weeks after finding all this out, I had had a conversation with my son about what was happening. He wanted me to forgive my husband. I was really shocked that he thought I could forgive that soon, and I was hurt that he wasn't supporting my side of things. I was taking a firm stance: I was right, and my husband was wrong. My son's request seemed totally unjustified and made me even more upset.

After talking to my son that night, and then having a terrible blow up with my husband, I had felt wretched — about as bad as I've ever felt. The pain in my heart was what I thought a heart attack would feel like, but I knew it was my heart breaking. I had said terrible things when we argued and been so mad that I'd had no filter for what I'd said. I had gone to bed totally spent, feeling absolutely awful. I laid awake a long time. "God, please help me with this. I'm in so much pain!" I cried and prayed and begged for another way, and eventually I'd fallen asleep.

The next morning, I woke up and started to write in my journal — doing what I always do. I didn't feel any different. I had a headache from all the crying. I was kind of groggy and going through my morning motions. I didn't write in my journal, though. Strangely, without thinking, I got a piece of paper and I started writing a letter — "Dear..." and then I realized I wasn't feeling like myself.

I became aware that I was in my husband. I was actually in his body and feeling his feelings. I knew that this was not my body because the feelings were completely unexpected and foreign. I noticed emotions that I knew were not mine, because I hadn't felt them before — not in the same way. It was so strange and entirely understandable at the same time. I never questioned what was happening even though it was so alien.

I could have been dreaming, but I was sitting up writing a letter while it was happening. I didn't know how to grasp the physiology of this — the phenomena of inhabiting someone else could be disturbing at best, but I didn't feel anything but wonder. It also felt familiar, because it was my husband, and although I hadn't known what he was thinking, my heart could see it was him.

I felt this overwhelming feeling of sadness, and maybe even more so of loneliness. The feeling of loneliness was excruciating. We hadn't had a good marriage in years and I recognized that loneliness, because it was similar to my own — but it was different, too. I felt his desperation and the yearning to be understood and loved: his sense of confusion at how things had gone so wrong when he was doing what he thought was the right thing to do. I knew at that moment that he had tried to do the right thing with the house but couldn't. There was great shame in his body. I had never experienced shame like this. Also, there was a sense of guilt so deep that it was completely unknown to me. I recognized the feeling of his heart breaking just like mine.

He was feeling worthless, and so I felt that, too — in my body. I felt feelings that have never been a part of me at all. I knew what they were, but I'd never experienced them before. But that was the gift; I did face it and feel it. The pain was very real. My sense of his pain connected to my pain, and, as I connected to these feelings and emotions, I felt my compassion swell.

As my compassion grew, I was able to understand the motivation, his rationalization, and saddest of all, the magnitude of his sense of failure. This all took place in a few minutes at most. It was all folded in on itself like I had been downloaded instantly with all the reasons and feelings he had. I couldn't pinpoint any of it or single out a certain moment. It seemed to have all transpired in a single gush of information inside my mind and body.

I sat there for a moment, trying to digest, but it was so complete that I didn't really need to make sense of it. It was very clear after it happened. Because of that, I wrote to him. I forgave him for everything. I told him I was so sorry too — sorry for whatever my part was in all of this, sorry for his pain and for my anger. I was sorry that we had both been so lonely in our marriage. I cried as I wrote about the years together and how I wouldn't trade our history.

I wrote about our family and how blessed we were to have what we had had — our beautiful kids and the twenty-five years of being married. I asked him to forgive me. I told him I would try to let go of all my anger — that it was rooted in fear, and I was scared, but I would do my best.

And with that, the pain in my chest just vanished, and a feeling of lightness replaced it. There was nothing left of the crushing sensation around my heart. The morning was going on like nothing had changed. I kind of mentally came around and was astonished at the magnitude of what had happened. I finished writing the letter, and I realized that I'd been given proof of how miraculous forgiveness can be.

I could say that what happened that morning might have stemmed from the fact that I'd had enough of feeling bad, and I wanted to stop the pain. I could say that I wanted my son to see me doing the right thing, so he would think better of me. Also, I might have wanted to forgive my husband just to validate what I'd been practicing for the last three years. But that wasn't true. I didn't want to forgive him — I hadn't been ready.

I had wanted him to feel the kind of pain that he "made" me feel. A part of me wanted to inflict as much pain on him as he had given me. This was old behavior, and I'd so easily slipped right back into it. I had been so far from feeling compassion for the situation — at that time, it had been beyond me.

I couldn't have gotten to forgiveness that morning from where I was the night before. There is no way. My son put the idea into my head to think about it, but I couldn't accept the idea. I was still rigid with anger.

I was still thinking of ways to hurt him until I felt his heart breaking too. How else could I have had the sympathy for him? The compassion came with the total understanding of being in his body and in what other way could I have gotten there in my angry condition? I don't know how long it would have taken to forgive him without sharing his pain and looking from inside him. Months? Years? Or maybe never.

My prayers the night before were heard, and I was given the gift of feeling my husband's pain, so I could let it all go. And I did. It was an amazing gift. What happened was an answered prayer, and when it happened, I recognized it for what it was. The gift of being in his body, the miracle of it, changed how I felt forever.

Although it all began with my cancer diagnosis, the proof of what I believe in came during my heartbreak. Prayers are heard, but more importantly, your heart needs to be in the right place to ask for another way. I think my broken heart was painful enough for me to reach out that night — to pray and be open to what might come. I believe that I opened up to goodness when I learned I had cancer, and it stayed with me. The foreclosure papers were on such a grand scale that I almost forgot what I'd learned until I prayed for another way.

What happened with my husband three years after my diagnosis is nothing short of amazing. I never would have been able to do what I did on my own. And, thankfully, I didn't have to. I prayed for help. Forgiving — true, absolute forgiveness — is life changing, and that's what I learned was possible. To ask for help with pain and to be open to receive another way is how our prayers are answered.

During the three years prior, I found the experiences, books, places, and friendships that helped me grow. It happened amazingly fast, that's true. Fundamental change takes time, but getting cancer puts you on the fast track if you let it. Doing things differently and being able to gather the courage to discover uncharted territory can become a way of life. It became what I looked for.

– 2 –
The Beginning

In 2010, I went to my doctor for a checkup, and she looked at me in shock when she felt the lump on my breast. I told her that I had it checked last year, and they had said it was a cyst. My doctor was adamant that I go that week for another scan — I was due for my mammogram anyway.

I had felt a lump in my right breast for years. In 1995, I discovered it and had a lumpectomy. It was a scary time for me. My mother had recently died of cancer, and with the family history, I thought for sure I was in trouble. But, as it ended up, they couldn't identify it as cancer, so it was left undetermined, and it was probably fibroids.

I felt the lump in the shower all the time. I got used to it. I was told after my mammogram in 2009 that I had a cyst there — so now it wasn't fibroids. Maybe that should have been a warning sign, but I didn't really care if it wasn't cancer. They did some more tests to be sure that it wasn't breast cancer. Apparently, it was just a cyst.

To be honest, I was a month late with my mammogram. I had a gyno appointment in December, and I should have had my mammogram in December, too. I didn't think it would be irresponsible to wait another month — what can happen in a month? So my doctor scheduled a mammogram that week. My doctor arranged for it "STAT," because she was so concerned.

After the mammogram, they took me to another room to have another kind of scan. I still wasn't too worried; after all, I had it checked last year. After waiting in there for at least an hour, a kind of dread began to crawl down my neck and back and landed as a queasy feeling in my gut. *I thought it was a cyst! It was, wasn't it? I had it checked out last year, and they SAID it was a cyst.* I kept trying to rationalize, but the realization was dawning on me that I might be in serious trouble here.

Finally, the door opened, and it was the radiologist, not the nurse. She asked the tech to give us some privacy. She looked me in the eye and was about to talk when, suddenly, I knew what she was going to say. At that moment, when she looked at me, I had seen it in her eyes that I did not have a cyst anymore. She had to look away, because she saw that I had understood. I had cancer.

I saw that she wished it weren't true; she seemed saddened by it. Legally, she couldn't tell me anything. She didn't say anything other than, "You will be getting a biopsy done this coming Tuesday at Woman and Infant's Hospital. This is not something you can put off." And with that, I got my clothes on and left — in a state of shock. I didn't need the biopsy to know. Her eyes had said it all.

There is no turning back once you know. Once you know, you're already stuck with it, and there's no way out…even if you want to postpone appointments or postpone thinking about it. You can't deny it and you can't run away. You're there and there's no turning around or pretending that your life will ever be the same. It's unfortunately your turn.

I went for the biopsy the next week. I knew what it would tell me. It's an uncomfortable procedure. It's the beginning of a long line of procedures. The operation itself is pretty quick, and I could be brave — I wasn't tired of it yet. I knew it was the first in a long line of hospital beds, and at that point, I had adrenaline keeping me focused.

I knew it would be a long haul, but I never thought that it would take as long as people told me. I didn't believe them. There may be people in your inner circle who have had cancer. You'll tell them you're going in for a biopsy. They'll give you advice and put you in their prayers. They'll tell you how long this will take, and you won't believe them, because that would be a year of your life! You'll wait and see, because it might be different for you. I was pretty sure I was going to get done with it much quicker, but that wasn't the case.

After the biopsy, you play the waiting game, pretending that you can concentrate on anything else — you wait. If you're like me, you're already planning how this will all go down. I used to be a big planner. I could plan months out, years out, thinking I had control over my future. I was never good at waiting, but this is one time you'll get pretty good at it. You'll have a lot of practice by the time it's over. My planning never made a bit of difference. I couldn't control the huge system that deals with breast cancer. It doesn't care about your schedule.

The cancer center where I had chosen to go was a large building with many doctors, therapists, and nurses. They worked in teams, and they met once a month to discuss your case. I highly recommend a group that's all connected. It was well organized and made me realize that this was happening to a LOT of people. The waiting room had at least seventy-five chairs in it.

My husband went with me, and we sat there in silence, waiting to be called in. What can you say to each other when you're at that kind of place? Silence is better than small talk at times like that. I had hopes that it would be just a little cancer — maybe we caught it early? There's always hope. I kept thinking of all the things they could say. I was trembling and sick to my stomach. I remember that I couldn't keep anything in me — lots of trips to the bathroom. My body had been in shock for a week now. You wake up in the morning and feel fine, and then it hits you like a brick, "Oh, God, I forgot — I have cancer."

No matter how much you think you're prepared, you're probably not.

This appointment is one that changes your life and what you thought you had — safety, security, health — what you thought you could control is now out of the question. Nobody asks for this kind of cataclysmic change, but for some of us, it comes. The big moment comes, and the question is not "whether" I can handle it, because I have to — the question becomes "how" will I handle this? The best part is that I get to choose how it goes. I can be beautiful or I can get stuck in myself. It's all a choice.

> "Hardship often prepares an ordinary person for an extraordinary destiny."
>
> — C.S. Lewis

The nurse showed us to a little room, and we waited there. They didn't ask me to undress. Clearly, we were just going to talk. That could be good, I thought. So after about twenty minutes, a doctor walked in and introduced himself. He started talking about what kind of treatments were available and what they had to offer, and I asked, "Wait, do I have cancer?"

He answered, "Of course, that's why you're here."

My ears started buzzing, and I couldn't focus — apparently, my shock was just kicking in. I was feeling sick, and I was trying to hold myself steady, and he's just talking and talking. So I started to say something, trying to get a word in and he said, "Just let me finish." He seriously said that. Like what he was saying was so much more important than what I had to say. The fact that he'd just told me that I had breast cancer kind of passed over like it was a given — which to me it wasn't — and he wanted to talk about what HE was going to do. I hopped off the table and left the room while he was in mid-sentence.

It's a good thing I didn't have a gown on, because I would have walked right out anyway. All along, I had had the feeling that the news would be what I was hearing — but when it came right down to it, I wasn't prepared. I still needed the time to digest the fact.

I went to a little open living room across the hall where you're supposed to go when you need to fall apart. And I fell apart. I started to cry, and I called my youngest sister. I said, "I have breast cancer," and then I had to hang up. A therapist was there within minutes.

I told her that the doctor was definitely not for me, and I couldn't possibly work with him. She was great, and she said she could get me the phone numbers of the other hospitals in the area if I wanted to go somewhere else. I thought that was very kind of her. She won me over.

I tried to calm myself — breathe, Kim, take a breath — and by then my husband had left the doctor and come to sit with me. A very nice woman in a white coat came and sat next to me. I assumed she was a doctor, but I didn't know. She was pretty, and I liked her shoes. She was calm and kind, and she wasn't talking — she was listening. I liked her a lot. She told me her name, and I remembered that was the same name someone had given me — they said she was the best surgeon I could ask for.

So right there, I said, "Will you be my doctor?" she said, "Of course." So just like that, it all began.

By the end of the year, I would be so happy to have run into her that day. She was a choice I made from my heart, and I never regretted it. I loved her whole way of being. That's what you want when you pick someone who's going to take pieces of you...someone who's really right for you.

There are a lot of things to do in the beginning. The way I handled it was to listen to my options, get opinions from doctors and friends who knew about what I was going through, trust my gut to decide, and then completely let it go. Make decisions and then leave it to the professionals. You can do research forever on what you have and still come out in the same place. You can second guess the hospital, the doctors, the clinicians — but it becomes a matter of where you want to spend your time and your energy.

The trick is to be able to let it go — once you've picked your team, you trust them to do their job, and then you work on what you're responsible for, which is your attitude and what you believe. I remembered it wasn't the situation I was in that mattered; it was what I did with it. I learned what I needed to do as I went. I trusted my instincts, and they inevitably led me to the most important year of my life. They led me past the cancer into a future I never would have dreamed for myself. Letting go of the details is something that I learned to do in general. Trust that you are going to be led and believe that the course you're on is the right one.

15

There is a pervasive attitude in fighting cancer. The war on cancer. Battling cancer. I chose to think of it as something to be faced with strength, but kindness too. I didn't want to be at war with my body. Although part of me was pretty upset that my body had gotten sick without my conscious permission, I wasn't going to fight against the cancer — I was going to work with my body. I didn't want a battle — I just wanted to get better.

"Fighting," "battling," and "warring" were not the words I wanted to use in connection with my illness.

It didn't feel right. I wanted cooperation, caring, understanding, and compassion for my body. I wanted to work WITH my body — love the sick parts back to health and believe in my healing. My fear became the energy that fueled the fire to get well, but the thought behind the fear was based on nurturing. I gained a profound purpose for my life — a shocking shift in my perspective, and maybe for first time, I became truly focused.

Everyone will react differently when they are diagnosed with cancer. You don't know how it'll go — you can't plan it. I had no way of knowing that I'd be happier after the experience. It didn't happen all at once. I wasn't happy that I had cancer. I was really scared about the whole thing, but I was somehow able to focus that fear. I wasn't good just sitting with my fear — although I would try. I had to put my energy somewhere.

– 3 –
A No-Brainer

Although looking at my diet was the first thing I did when I found out I had cancer, it was not the most important thing. Had I known what I know now, I probably would have started working on my thoughts before anything else. Not knowing it was also part of my journey. Changing my diet was kind of a no-brainer, pardon the pun, because having the power to change my thoughts was not something I understood yet. Being aware of how my opinions effected every aspect of my health and life had to come a little later.

This chapter on diet is important, but only from the body's perspective. I begin with it because it's how I began — with what I knew I could do. Controlling my mind was not something that I'd ever considered before, but it is way beyond what you choose to put into your body. With that said, what you eat, how you eat, and why you eat are all directly affected by your feelings about food. If you can approach eating in general with a positive attitude and believe that your efforts will help you achieve optimum health, you will greatly improve your body's own abilities. It's all in your point of view.

When I was told I had cancer, I immediately thought of what I could do right away. Our diet is probably the first thing most of us think about when we think about changing our health. What have I been putting in my body that might have contributed to my cancer? There is so much out there that you can be scared of eating. We know about all the chemicals on and in the soil that grow the vegetables and fruits available to us. We know about all the unpronounceable additives in the packaged food we're able to buy. Hopefully, we know enough about nutrition to keep trans fats, refined sugars and grains, and processed and fast food to a minimum, but looking honestly at what we're putting into our bodies is a very beneficial way to focus your attention, especially if you're not well. If you are what you eat, that should make you feel good, not worried.

I changed a lot of what I was eating, and although the diet I followed may seem radical to some, I did a huge amount of research. I felt that my diet needed to be extreme, because that's what my body was telling me to do — it made perfect sense to me. I highly recommend doing what makes sense to you. It's what your mind attaches to it that will make a difference. All the information is out there, and its ongoing — new information is available all the time on what our bodies need and want. Decide what sounds right to you and apply it.

I'm not encouraging you to do exactly as I did, but to listen to what your body wants.

– 4 –
Creative Recovery

I spent hours and hours a day doing Internet searches, reading books, making special food, seeing doctors, and asking advice. My question was always the same: "What more can I do to help my body heal? Food, exercise, rest, books, research, water, laughter — you name it — Reiki, yoga, meditation, journaling, coffee enemas, smoothies.... I did whatever it took to keep me actively involved in my recovery. If it sounded good to me, I'd try it. If it didn't feel right, I'd stop.

The eating regimen that I chose to follow was of my own, and it made sense to me. I put together a lot of different ideas from different places. It took a lot of time — sometimes hours — to prepare food for a few days. This seemed to calm me. It was part of my job. I had to have a program for myself that showed I was doing all I could to help me heal.

I have had years and years of training regarding food — nothing official, but training nonetheless. Obsessive and compulsive behaviors surrounding my eating had me doing lots of research and reading for forty years. I remember when I was twelve, in the '70s,

I decided to become a vegetarian, and I went out to the yard every day and picked dandelion greens (it drove my mother crazy). Since then I've been pretty serious about what went into my body, believing that what I ate was a part of me. I had been eating lots of raw food, growing organic produce, and foraging for greens for years and years — so this "new" diet was not really a stretch for me. Most of us who've been driven (or compulsive) about nutrition and food have a database of knowledge that could be turned into volumes.

I was thirty-three when my mother died of cancer. I looked very closely at the way we ate as a family after that — my kids were one and two years old — and it wasn't easy to eat mostly vegetables, but whole food was a must. Cooking from scratch takes a lot of time, but at least you know where your ingredients come from. I still had a lot of room for improvement. I knew that my diet hadn't been the cause of my cancer, but it was something to focus on, and it helped me feel positive and proactive. If I could make changes that I knew were going to be beneficial, I'd do it.

My way of thinking at that time was that if I had been doing it before, and I got cancer, then it would be advantageous to change it now that I was going to get better. That meant changing a lot. It might seem crazy to change so much, but I WAS a little crazy. I was very serious and determined to improve my health and well-being any way that I could.

When my eating routine and diet shifted, it gave me a lot to do, and that was just what I needed. I required a job to keep my mind busy from thinking fearful or negative thoughts. All the work that went into making my food was concentrated, positive energy. My job was now to get better, and I put everything I had into it. That concentrated energy could have been the shift that helped my health the most. I made it fun. I enjoyed it. I loved making the food, and even more, eating it. I was happy with the purpose behind it. I felt confident that I was making a difference and helping my body.

That appointment for my mammogram, when I looked into the radiologist's eyes, was the day I stopped eating three-quarters of what I had been eating for the last ten years. I had not yet received a diagnosis, but as I said, I had a feeling what was about to happen, and I quit drinking coffee and alcohol, and stopped eating white sugar, white flour, dairy, eggs, and anything that had eyes without even knowing the outcome of the biopsy. It happened that fast. The panic — "What can I do to help me heal?" — took over and pushed me into action. My body knew and I went along with it. The research came later.

The reason for these choices was, at some very rudimentary level, I knew that what I needed was what my body was telling me — I had a gut feeling, and I responded to that. What my body wanted was whole food — nothing refined and nothing cooked. I was listening to my body, not my emotions. I also really believed what my body was telling me, which is very important. If you are going to choose to follow a special diet, the only way that it'll be really helpful is if you believe in it. If you dislike what you're eating and you're following a program because you've been told to, it won't help you.

Only foods that were alive and all organic were going into my mouth. The body craves what vegetables have to offer when you take habit and emotional eating out of the picture. Vegetables are the builders of the body, and fruits are the cleaners of the body. Yes, of course, we need protein, and animals are a great way to get it, but they aren't necessarily healthy for all of us all the time. When I was choosing what my body wanted when it needed to heal, animals were not on the menu.

– 5 –
Alkaline Diet

A fter quite a bit of research, I decided to concentrate on a raw diet. The main reason why raw was on my radar was because of alkalinity. The alkalinity of vegetables and fruits is just one of the benefits of eating live foods — vitamins, minerals, fiber, and enzymes are all available in live foods. There is a lot of information about cancer loving an acidic environment. Cancer actually creates an acidic environment, but I thought that changes to bring my alkalinity up would be very helpful. Again, it made sense to me, and what made sense seemed to be what my body wanted.

Alkaline foods help the blood hold more oxygen — up to 100 times more than in an acidic environment. Too much acidity in the body creates a toxicity that is unhealthy and can lead to disease. Cancer thrives in acid. That was all I needed to hear — that and an alkaline diet is all about vegetables and fruits. An acidic environment is created by sugars, animal products, refined grains, processed foods, coffee, soda, and alcohol.

The point of making your body more alkaline is not to be totally alkaline — that's not good either — it's about balance. The aim is to be more alkaline than acidic. Eating more raw vegetables will automatically shift your chemistry, but the degree to which you do that is up to you. There are lots of little things you can do to shift your chemistry in the right direction. If you're working towards keeping your system more alkaline, a few things you can do will make a big difference.

Remember that being happy and living your life is absolutely more important than your diet.

If you have habits that could use a little tweaking, think about everything in moderation and be comfortable with your new choices. There are lists on the Internet for acidic and alkaline foods, but they are not all the same. Personally, I feel that adding more fruits and vegetables to your diet is always a good way to start, whether they are listed as acid-forming or not; they're still better than potato chips and soda. Here's a few places to start:

- This has nothing to do with your diet, but this is something you should be aware of: stress and worry will create an acidic environment in your body. This is good to know, especially when you might be worried about your health — try to keep your stress levels to a minimum and stop worrying. Do the best you can and then let it all go.

- Switch your morning coffee to green tea or try herbal coffee. (It's really good) Decaf is just as acidic as regular, so cutting back on coffee or getting rid of it as a habit makes a difference.
- Drink lemon with your water. Water can be acidic, and adding lemon to it makes it more alkaline.
- Edit out soda from your day — think of it as a very special treat.
- Eat more vegetables.
- Eat more fruits.
- Soak nuts in salt water, and then dehydrate them at 115 degrees.
- Lessen or eliminate all processed foods, white flour, white sugar, red meat, and alcohol.

I changed my eating habits overnight, and my family went along with this amazingly well. They ate the same things they usually ate, but when it came to me making dinner every night, we all ate the same. Eating mostly raw can be very delicious, but it was totally different than what we we're used to. I think they were all just trying to do their part in supporting me. And while they felt they were helping me, it gave us all something else to concentrate on. It sure gave us a lot to talk about.

I was eating only living things, and it was obvious something was different — I was visibly changing. My skin was smoother. I could see better (I actually didn't need my glasses as much). I felt amazing and looked so much healthier. When I looked in the mirror, I saw sparkles in my eyes; my eyelids weren't puffy at all, and it made me look younger. The lines and wrinkles on my face visibly shrunk, and my complexion looked clearer. By the time I had my first surgery to put my port in, I had been asked by at least four people what I was doing to look so good. They didn't know that I had been diagnosed with cancer, but it was that noticeable in just a few weeks.

I shopped all the time for produce — maybe every three days. Luckily, I had a Whole Foods and year-round farmers markets near me, as well as my own garden when the weather warmed up. When you're only eating organic and raw, it has to be very fresh because taste becomes paramount. I was adding to my compost pile morning, noon, and night. My friends were bringing me books on raw, and one of my friends gave me a dehydrator and a Vitamix blender — quite a gift! A lot of work was spent preparing the food, but it was all worth the effort.

There are many books on eating raw. Some of my favorites are: *Living Cuisine* by Renee Loux Undercoffler, *Fresh* by Sergei and Valya Boutenko, *Rawvolution* by Matt Amsden, and *The Complete Idiot's Guide to Eating Raw* by Mark Reinfield, Bo Rinaldi, and Jennifer Murray. Raw eating can be quite gourmet, but that's a stretch for the average cook. As long as you have a wide variety of vegetables, fruits, sprouted seeds, and soaked nuts, your nutrition should be fine. I stayed away from soy products except edamame. A good organic whey protein powder with almond milk for added protein in your diet would be very beneficial.

The whole point of raw eating is that the food still has its enzymes intact. When you cook food, the heat kills the enzymes and lots of the vitamins. Enzymes start to die at about 118 degrees. Most cooking is way above that. All raw vegetables, nuts, seeds, grains, and fruits have their own enzymes. Anything alive has enzymes. Enzymes will work on digesting what they're found in — so, in other words, the enzymes in an apple will help digest that apple. Your body doesn't need to add to it. This leaves the body's enzymes that you normally use to digest foods for use another time. Keeping all the enzymes alive helps your body by doing the work and storing all the vitamins and minerals available for you. Basically, what you're eating takes care of itself and puts less pressure on the body to perform the act of assimilating the food.

You are what you eat — at least on a physical level. What you consume becomes your body. Putting food that doesn't help you into your mouth is something that needs to be weighed: *"Is this going to be so tasty that I don't care that it's not nourishing?"* When you're sick, and your body needs help to get back to its normal healthy self, you might want to ask yourself that question. *"Do I really have to have this piece of cake?"* If the answer is absolutely 'yes,' then eat it with a smile on your face, and think about how amazing it tastes and how good it is. Stressing about what you eat doesn't do anything but make what could be a good experience a wasted one.

On the other hand, if you're going to expect your diet to help change what's happening in your body, there has to be some sort of compromise. If you feel strongly that a certain diet will help you, be realistic about how well you're following it. It doesn't have to be forever — it can last for as long as it takes for your body to respond. I would say at least a few months to see a change in your health. I went six months on the raw diet, and then I began to add some animal protein. I continued to stay with the rest of it, but I had given it a block of time to work.

A typical day would look something like this:

Breakfast: Green smoothie with kale, Swiss chard, one peeled lemon, half of a banana and a knob of ginger, and 12 –18 ounce of pure water

Midmorning: homemade granola with raw nuts, oats, seeds, and fruit

Lunch: Salad of chopped kale, avocado, red pepper, shredded carrots, pea pods, cilantro, sunflower seeds, and sprouts, raw cider vinegar and olive oil

Midafternoon: Apple with raw almond butter

Dinner: Spiralized zucchini "pasta" with cashew cream, and peach pie with raw walnut and agave crust

Juicing always seemed to be a bit of a waste to me, because you get none of the natural fiber — I believe the body should have all that fiber that juicing takes away. The beauty of juicing is that it's taken into your body immediately — there is no need for digesting. Your body doesn't have to do much to absorb all the vitamins and minerals. The drawback of juicing is that it's high in sugar and most juices should be diluted with water. With that said, I occasionally juiced beets, ginger, and carrots, which are hard to do in a blender.

Making smoothies with lots of vegetables was my go-to for breakfast and in between meals. The difference between juicing and smoothies is that one is nothing but juice and the other is all of the fruit and vegetables blended in a blender. I drank at least 30 ounces of green smoothie every day. I would make a blender full and carry it around with me until I finished it. It was mostly kale and Swiss chard (mainly because that's what I had growing in my garden), but I would add a chunk of ginger, a peeled whole lemon, dandelion greens, and anything else I could find in my garden. I added half a banana when I needed something sweeter.

Also, I did quite a bit of foraging. I bet you're wondering what that is — "foraging." I would use the edible weeds from my garden for eating and smoothies — what I could find in and around my yard (don't laugh). You would be surprised at the nutrition levels of most "weeds." The difference in the vitamin content is significant in foraged greens. I had been doing this since I was a kid when I read you could eat weeds. You should be certain of the plant you plan to eat. Until you get used to the look of a plant, make sure you know what it is. There are lots of books on foraging and plenty of information on the Internet. The plants vary depending on where you live, but they're available – just go look at your garden.

I would daily add dandelion, red clover, purslane, wood sorrel, and lamb's quarters to my smoothies. These weeds grew right in my garden! I finally started appreciating them for what they were giving me in nutrition and letting them grow instead of "weeding" to get rid of them. Make sure you don't eat anything that you've used chemicals or fertilizers on — organic is the aim for everything that goes into your mouth.

I eat bunches of flat leaf parsley and cilantro every week. Cilantro is a natural chelator, which means it binds to metals in your body, and then carries them out. Herbs are a great way to get flavor and vitamins into your diet. Chervil is delicious when you can find it and easy to grow. Dill, basil, and sorrel are also good in salads.

Although greens and raw vegetables are the main part of my diet, I also eat a lot of raw, soaked nuts that I then dehydrate. Sprouting grains and seeds and soaking nuts rids them of phytic acid and enzyme inhibitors. When you soak nuts and sprout seeds, you greatly reduce the acid in them. Soak nuts for at least six hours, with some sea salt added to the water. When you've rinsed them, put them in a dehydrator at 118 degrees until they're crunchy again. Now the nuts have much less acid and their enzymes are available, so you can digest them much easier.

The only drawback of raw that I can see is that you are forever looking for that certain "crunch." I can make a mean cracker in the dehydrator, but it can't hold a candle to a regular rice cracker. Although I still eat a lot of raw, I now eat yogurt, cheese, animal protein, and rice crackers! Other than that, I follow the same "diet" as when I started.

Variety in your diet is more important than you might think. Make a conscious effort to eat lots of different vegetables and fruits and try to eat a lot of foods raw. It's common knowledge that dark leafy greens are the best vegetables, but eating all kinds is the key to getting optimum vitamins: kale and chard, Brussel sprouts, cabbage, spinach, arugula, dandelion greens, beet greens, and all kinds of herbs, to name a few.

Everything should be organic when you can find it — there's no question about it. The only things I will eat that aren't organic are veggies and fruits that have a thick rind or skin that you can cut off — and this doesn't always work. Apples have been found to have pesticides in their flesh, which, I'm sure, is true for other fruits and vegetables, so peeling them isn't the issue. It's what's in the ground that goes into the plant when it gets watered.

There is a list that comes out every year called the "dirty dozen," and this list is what I avoid; I will only buy organic. These are the fruits and veggies that are the most tainted with chemicals. It's usually soft fleshed fruits — peaches, plums, berries, and the vegetables range every year. I've heard that industrial potato farmers won't eat their own crops. Pay attention to the dirty dozen. You don't want your body to have to defend itself from what you eat! Support organics by using your dollar as your voice.

I believe that animals carry the same kind of energy that we do. If I am going to eat an animal and put it into my body, I'm going to do my best to eat one that has been treated humanely. If it's going into my body, to the best of my ability, I won't eat something that has suffered being raised to feed me. I treat my body with respect and also the things I eat.

When you start to put your money literally where your mouth is, it makes a difference in how you eat. Buying an animal that has been humanely raised is very expensive! When you pay double for the meat you're eating because it was treated humanely, you cook it differently and eat it differently. What you spend alone for it will change how you feel about consuming it.

If you're paying attention to what your body's telling you, avoid anything that makes you feel uncomfortable. Most often, this will mean that you're eating certain foods together that don't digest well when combined. Very rarely will a raw vegetable make you uncomfortable, but eating it with lots of other foods might upset your stomach. Don't eat foods that are "good" for you that your body doesn't digest well. Just because it's good for people, doesn't mean it's for "you" specifically. You are an individual, and your diet should be yours. Respect the cues you get from your body and listen!

Lots of people have food issues. We all have things that we eat, because we like the taste or how it fills our emotional need, but it might not make our bodies happy. If you have chronic problems with indigestion, bloating, or constipation, try looking at your diet from your body's perspective. Don't eat things just because you're used to eating them. You can figure out what it is that's making you uncomfortable by starting very simply with what you know is okay and adding foods one at a time. If you're really serious about feeling better, start a journal and keep a food log. The minute you feel a reaction, look at what you ate last and keep track of what that was. Eventually, you can eliminate the foods that don't make your body happy.

I have a gluten sensitivity. It took me a long time to figure it out. I wasn't focused on the problem; I would just feel bloated and gassy and generally out of sorts for years! Eventually, I got tired of feeling crappy and I really put some effort into figuring out what was wrong. I tried giving up things one at a time. I was so surprised to find that so many totally unrelated things gave my body a hard time. Garlic, chocolate, cornmeal, wheat, peanuts, and eggs all are hard on my system. Sometimes if you stay away from a food that bothers you for a couple of months, you can eat small amounts every so often without any reaction.

When I asked the nutritionist at the hospital what kind of diet she would recommend, I was really taken aback. The nutritionist at the cancer center was quite young, and I would have thought very "up-to-date" with what I consider to be what's "now" in food. That was not the case at all. I felt like I was looking at a food plan from a 1980s weight-watcher meeting. Don't just listen to what a nutritionist tells you — trust yourself — *you will know what's right*. Do some research and decide what you think sounds good to your body. Trust your instincts.

The suggestions from a holistic doctor would be good if you don't want to make your own food choices. The American diet is not easy on your system — I think we all know that by now — and your body needs all the help you can give it.

– 6 –
Eating with Attitude

When I followed my own plan, I had incredible energy, I slept better, I looked younger than I had in years, I lost weight — which was never the intent, but I felt my body was happier than it had ever been, and I was so grateful. I gave my body a chance to work on itself and begin healing. I wasn't eating anything that taxed my system. My body thanked me all day long.

Denying yourself something you really want can be very uncomfortable and feel like a form of punishment. If you absolutely want something, don't deny yourself. Whether you really want it or not is the interesting part. It's just so easy to listen to your inner child. Will what you want nourish you? Will you feel guilt or pleasure once you've had it? What's the best for your overall health, and can you be grown-up enough to get to the bottom of that question? How healthy do you want to be? How much do you love your body?

Denial is not the goal here; not at all. The goal is to feel so great that you want to eat the way your body is directing you. And the diet that you follow can be all your own. If you are successful in eating what your body wants, you'll feel wonderful. Separating what YOU want from what your body wants isn't the easiest because of all the years of eating for pleasure and emotional need. What you may find is that the healthier you eat, the more your body recognizes and craves what is good for it. You have to give it a chance to feel the benefits (weeks, maybe months), and after that, old habits and cravings will fall away for the most part. I still like chocolate, but I don't eat it all the time because even if I like it, my body does not. Once your body has a "taste" of what it needs, it'll want more. I have had my mouth water while I'm picking weeds to put in my smoothie - honestly.

When you are eating, you can make a practice of honoring what you are putting into your body and honoring yourself for the attention you're giving yourself. By honoring, I mean taking a moment to recognize what you're doing and being grateful. If you're putting all this effort into your food, you should be very happy that you're helping your body heal. Be thankful for what's in front of you. You can also take a moment to recognize that what you're about to put into your mouth is exactly what you need at the moment, and you've decided it's what your body wants. Trust yourself and your choices. You know yourself better than anybody else — be happy and sure that you're doing everything right.

One of the best books I've ever read about eating and what we attach to food is *Woman Food and God,* written by Geneen Roth. She uses the following guidelines for eating that could be used by everyone for mindfulness:

1. Eat when you are hungry.
2. Eat sitting down in a calm environment.
3. Eat without distractions. Distractions include radio, TV, newspapers, books, intense or anxiety provoking conversations or music.
4. Eat what your body wants.
5. Eat until you are satisfied.
6. Eat (with the intention of being) in full view of others.
7. Eat with enjoyment, gusto, and pleasure.

I don't go crazy if my plans are thwarted and I can't eat organic, or if I don't have any healthy options for a particular meal. I stay relaxed and remember that my attitude about the food is more important than the food itself. Being grateful and truly happy about what you're about to eat is much more beneficial to you than the most healthy meal. A grateful heart is the best emotion to be feeling when you're eating. Breathe, slow down, and taste your food — slow down and love what you're eating.

If I take an extra hour to make my lunches up for the next three or four days, and I know that it's really wholesome, organic produce that my body needs and likes digesting, I will feel excellent eating it, and it will make a difference in how I feel on the inside. Your body is amazingly wise, with a natural tendency toward good health — helping your body by listening closely will greatly improve your health. When you're dealing with an illness, try not to tax your body. Give it pure, organic food, lots of water, and rest. Eat carefully while you recover — once you're feeling better and have healed, then you can relax your program, and only if it feels good to change.

Above all, listen to what your body says it wants, not what you want just because it gives you an emotional response. Try to separate the emotion from the food. There are times when eating for comfort is great, and we all need that, but when that becomes your normal behavior, you don't get the nutrition that your body needs. When you can separate the emotion from your food, for the most part, you have the ability to see what your body is asking for.

Your body is your sole responsibility, and you need to get to know it and work with it. Nobody else is going to put things in your mouth for you. Your body is not going to function at its best unless you pay attention to it, and it will thrive with attention. It will tell you what you need to know, but you also need to understand how to listen, so you will know the best way for you to eat. Changing your diet won't likely cure you in and of itself, but it can go a very long way to helping your overall health and well-being.

My new diet naturally gave my body a lot of help. Working on my food was something that I could do to take control and relieve stress. I would have my treatments, go home, and do my thing. I drank kale smoothies every day, read spiritual books, meditated, exercised outdoors, breathed deeply, and relaxed. My job was to concentrate on my healing and to bring as much love and attention to my body as possible.

– 7 –
Leave the Wine Behind

When my diet changed, so did the way I drank alcohol. I had been drinking a glass of wine or two a night for about thirty years. Alcohol was the way I relaxed, celebrated, killed time, enjoyed friends, de-stressed, cured boredom, and consoled myself.

I grew up in an alcoholic home. I learned early about the dangers and chaos caused by drinking, but that didn't stop me from doing it. I began drinking at an early age, and although I drank all the time, I was careful. The older I got, the more careful I became. I continued to drink, but I was always concerned and worried about my family history, so I'd stop after one or two drinks.

When I was in treatment for cancer, alcohol was the first thing on my list to go. My body said definitely "NO," so I listened. I became a nondrinker for the first time in my adult life. I had quit during my pregnancies, but this was a different kind of life change, because I knew it would be long term. I didn't think about it at the time, but it was another gift that cancer gave me. Giving up alcohol wasn't as hard as I thought it would be, because, at that time, I wanted to do anything that would increase my chances of full recovery.

I view my habitual drinking as something that held me back from my full potential. I spent years having a glass of wine every night. It wasn't until I had quit that I realized how much it sapped my energy and kept me from feeling clear. It helped me avoid doing what I could have been doing.

I am nowhere near my best when I drink. I'm not saying that drinking is bad, because it's not, but I spent so much time using it as a coping mechanism, that I lost sight of the downside of it. Escaping can be fun, but when it becomes a nightly thing, at least for me, it became a way to hide and pretend that I was together when I wasn't. I think that kind of "relaxing" is overrated.

Drinking as a habit is much different than choosing to have a drink. If it's part of a routine, you don't question whether you're going to have one or not. There's that time of the day when you pour yourself a drink — it's not a question. If it's something that's a very consistent part of your day, then you become so accustomed to it that you don't even think about it. When it becomes a ritual, it changes you. Maybe only slightly, but it does.

Habits become part of your character.

I have always had a complicated relationship with alcohol. My upbringing made sure of that. It wasn't the alcohol itself; it was what happened to the people around me when they drank. As a child, I was resentful of my mother's way of avoiding my needs in lieu of having a drink. It was about her copping out and ignoring what needed to be addressed in the name of a drink. Her concentrating on the act of drinking instead of connecting with me was what hurt — and it works that way for a lot of us.

In my adult life, I've had relationships with many people who drink as a habit. When drinking is habitual, the connection in the relationship often suffers. What happens is the drink becomes the focus, and it creates a disconnection between the people. The space between you widens every time you choose a cocktail over a genuine connection. It can be fun to drink with your spouse, family, or your friends, but when it's all the time, it's about numbing and avoiding, not connecting. It becomes damaging, because it's a way to avoid what might need to be paid attention to, whether it's uncomfortable, boring, or just the truth.

Some of the most painful memories in my life have been when someone I loved and needed chose to drink instead of stay with me. What I mean by "stay with me" is that they chose to drink instead of just be there — sober. This has happened all throughout my life with the people I have loved and cared about. They chose to have a drink instead of truly connecting. Drinking takes the edge off, it's true, but it becomes the primary focus instead of connecting with or paying attention to the people you love. I am just as guilty of doing this as anyone that's done it to me.

That's where my guilt comes in. I feel guilty choosing to check out instead of choosing to be available. Life is just too precious to be numbed for it — even the hard parts. It is very powerful to be truly present when you are relating to someone. It's as much a gift to you as the gift you're giving when you're fully there in the moment. Connecting when you're drinking is not the same. It's as though you're wearing an emotional coat. That barrier keeps your relationship at a distance.

I never would have been able to quit just for the sake of quitting. I didn't think I needed to. It was just a part of my life, and I didn't think it was a "bad" part, just one that I needed to be careful of. What I didn't know was the amount of baggage attached to it for me. I didn't understand this until I quit. I couldn't drink when I had cancer, because that would have gone against my whole plan. I had to quit, and I was grateful for the reason.

– 8 –
Pray for Peace

At the time I was diagnosed, I began to pray. That was pretty understandable, given the situation. What I prayed for was kind of obscure, though; I prayed for peace. I never even thought about it when I started doing it. Peace was kind of a strange thing to focus on for me — why not health or strength or courage? I could have used all of those, too, but peace was what came to me, so I prayed for that.

I wanted to feel peace, and I prayed every day. I wrote about peace, I asked for peace in my journal. I have written pages and pages for weeks on end about me seeking peace. Truthfully, I didn't know at the time what I meant by it. I didn't care; it was just what kept coming up. "Dear God, please bring me peace." From fear? Peace for my busy head? Peace in my heart, my life? I wasn't sure what I had meant, but I wrote it all the time anyway. What made me start to pray for it, I'll never know.

For me, to pray for peace before this whole transformation would have seemed ridiculous. I seriously would have laughed at it. In the past, the thought of peace was perhaps the farthest thing from my mind. What did I need peace for? Peace held no attraction for me because I was perpetually busy.

Busyness is a choice that doesn't include peace.

As the time went by without drinking, I realized I was seeing things in a different way. The clarity I was getting from not drinking alcohol was amazing. I couldn't believe the difference. I hadn't gone a month without a glass of wine in twenty years. It never occurred to me that it was going to affect the way I thought and the way I felt so profoundly. I thought maybe the fact that I was in chemotherapy was the reason I was feeling so different. I didn't put two and two together until after the chemo was over, and I continued to have this clear, light feeling. It dawned on me one day that this was peace I was feeling and it was because I wasn't drinking.

I felt a calmness that I wouldn't have attributed to getting rid of alcohol. You think of alcohol as something that calms you down, but that's not necessarily the case. It is a depressant, but it doesn't calm. It might slow you down, but it doesn't calm you. It diminishes your clarity. The peace that I felt when I quit a thirty-year habit is beyond explanation for me. I would wake up every morning with a sense of peace that was exponentially more than one glass of wine could have explained.

To date, cutting alcohol out of my life at that time has been one of the best changes I've ever made. It began with so much questioning for me, because I finally had the clarity to see what I needed to ask about. I discovered transparency where there was so much confusion. I became clear enough to discover me underneath all the hiding I was doing. Even having cancer wouldn't have woken me up to this extent, unless I had the lucidity to see the lessons.

I will never take for granted the peace of mind I get without alcohol. It doesn't have any power over me anymore; there's no habit. Alcohol is something that affects so many of us in so many ways. I never dreamt that I could love my life without it, or that my life would be so much better without the habit. I also never realized that it had such an influence on my way of living, my way of reacting, and my way of seeing things. It has been wonderful to find such great change with something so deceptively simple.

– 9 –
The Elixir of Life

C hanging your diet is very helpful, but if you could do only one thing that would change how your body functioned, it would be to drink more water. Adding water to my routine is the single most helpful thing that I've done for my body.

Obviously, with all the water for sale, we've been drinking it. It seems when people drink water, most of them think it has to be from plastic water bottles. The US consumed 50 BILLION water bottles last year — that's 1,500 bottles every second. Maybe it could be consumed in a reusable container? Please? Drinking water is a must for good health, but it doesn't have to be out of plastic bottles.

I was told to drink a lot of water when I was receiving chemo. Water dilutes the wastes and toxins that need to leave your body. The more water you can drink, the easier it is to flush your system. Any time you are taking a lot of medicines or have been sick, drinking water will help your body eliminate what it doesn't want or need. For the kidneys and liver to filter your blood and free toxins from it, water is very necessary. It's necessary for all of your organs to function properly.

I had started drinking more water when I changed my diet, and then more during chemotherapy, but I didn't really have a minimum amount or a formula until I started doing the research. Eight glasses of water is a good starting point, and that's something that we've always heard, but you have to actually do it for it to work for you.

The same amount of ounces as 60 percent of your body weight is what I've determined as a good rule of thumb. If you're taking lots of medication or going through chemo, you could add to that. If it's hot out, I'll drink more, and that does not count other liquids. If you weigh 130 pounds, that's about 80 ounces of water a day.

When you drink water it should be in small amounts at a time. Drinking large amounts all at once defeats the purpose and actually isn't good for you. The point is to keep you totally hydrated and to dilute the body's wastes and help all the body's functions go more smoothly. Your body can be as much as 60 percent water. It's estimated that 75 percent of Americans are chronically dehydrated. With 1,500 bottles bought every second? How is this possible?

We know we should drink, but we don't drink water. We drink coffee, lots of soda, alcohol, tea, energy drinks — something with taste or a buzz. Most of us have ignored our thirst for so long that we don't even feel it anymore. Once you've started drinking enough water to hydrate your body, you'll develop your thirst again.

Drinking a big glass of water right when you get up in the morning helps flush your system. After sleeping and being inactive, drinking hydrates you and wakes you up. It's also a great way to get a chunk of that water out of the way. My favorite way to get that morning hydration is to drink hot water with lemon, but it doesn't matter as long as you're drinking.

Also, I drink the juice of a whole lemon every day. Either as a hot tea with another ten ounces of water or added to one of my stainless steel containers. It helps flush the kidneys and liver. Lemon has an alkaline effect once it's in the body. Lemon water is very beneficial if you're working on an alkaline diet.

I usually juice three or four lemons, and then keep the juice in the fridge until I need it. When I'm filling up my water bottles in the morning, I'll put a big splash in my water and drink that all day. The vitamin C is excellent for you as well. I have two stainless steel 40-ounce containers that go everywhere with me. They don't break, and they are light and easy to throw in a backpack or the car.

You'll find that when you pay attention to your thirst, you don't really mind drinking all day. Lots of people say they want to drink eight glasses of water a day, but then breakfast comes and goes, and you have your coffee or tea and no water. Then lunch comes, and you haven't had more than a glass yet. You end up trying to fit all the water in for the day late in the afternoon. This is not the idea. Get a big container — preferably glass or stainless steel — and keep it with you all day long. Refill it when you run out.

– 10 –
Reading Your Body

I ignored my body's cues for most of my life. I actually took a certain pride in how much I could ignore them: how long I could work even when I was tired, how long I could put off going to the bathroom, how little sleep I could operate on, and, my personal favorite, how long I could go without eating or drinking. My natural thirst was something I never paid any attention to at all. In my case, it began as a form of self-abuse. I was unhappy with myself, and it made sense to ignore my needs. They weren't important.

When I was a teenager, I used to go all day without drinking anything (I thought that drinking would make me bloated) and all day without eating anything (I thought that eating would make me fat). I would do this for days and days. I wonder what my body thought was going on? The food and water were right there, but I ignored them and my body because of something I believed (no matter how stupid it was).

Neglecting my body never seemed like a big deal to me. I felt confident that I knew what was best. Nobody ever explained to me that my body knew what was best, and that's why we have thirst, hunger, fatigue, and pain. Funny how we can mess up such a perfect system and feel sure we're doing it better.

As I got older, I kept doing the same thing, only on a different level. We all do. We eat when we aren't hungry and don't drink when we're thirsty. We ignore pain and hope it goes away or take lots of pills to avoid feeling it. We don't get enough sleep, eat the wrong foods for our systems, keep working when we're overly tired and mentally spent, abuse drugs and alcohol, and live a sedentary lifestyle. We totally take for granted what our bodies are saying until we get sick. Getting sick will usually get your attention and can be a great wake-up call.

Your body is brilliant, and it knows exactly what to do to take care of itself. It doesn't hesitate. It's doesn't second guess. It's 100 percent competent and efficient. The problem is that "you" get in the way of it taking care of you. Your mind is the problem.

We have to learn how to heed our bodies' "warning system." It's not hard to hear what is being communicated if you give it a little attention. Listen to your body; don't wait until you get sick. If you have pain, a lump, a chronic condition, irritation — whatever it may be — figure it out. Work on it until you know what to do to fix it. Ask your body what it needs.

Your body is a neutral form on its own. Without your mind chiming in, it would be completely free of distractions and would operate with only one purpose: your total health and wellness. However, it has to work along with your mind; it has no choice. The two cannot be separated long enough to give your body a chance by itself. It responds to your thoughts all day, every day, every minute, and even while you sleep. It listens to what you assume to be true, and it knows what you believe — you can't fool it.

Your conscious and subconscious thoughts are directly linked to your body on every level. The body doesn't know the difference between what you actually experience and what you're thinking. We've all felt fear in a dream, and then woken up to see it isn't really happening, but it's the same fear that you have when you're awake. Your body can't distinguish between dreaming and being awake, and it responds to both in the same way. Imagining a scary situation is the same to the body as experiencing it in real time.

The body is completely unbiased without the mind to distract and reroute it. It works continuously to achieve balance and health. If we didn't have the mind putting its perceptions into the mix, the body would function with superior performance. Your body works very hard to maintain homeostasis. Homeostasis is what your body does to control your internal stability and keep bodily functions normal.

For every action, there is a reaction and regulation. For instance, if you get too hot, the body responds with sweat, and it starts to cool down. If you get an infection, your body responds with your immune system that fights unwanted micro-organisms. With over 150 trillion cells in the human body, chemical reactions are happening too fast to count, but they are all happening in accordance with each other for only our continued well-being.

The body is a direct reflection of the mind. Because it's neutral, it doesn't make any judgments — it leaves that to the mind. It will tell you everything you want to know and more. When you notice a pain somewhere, pay attention. You shouldn't notice anything when nothing is wrong. In other words, you shouldn't notice your throat unless it's sore. You don't notice a tooth until it hurts. When you have anything that feels off — aches, pains, trouble with your belly, your heart — look to your body for answers. Fix the things you can, such as going to a dentist when your tooth aches. But for chronic conditions, you might need to go within and start noticing what you're thinking about, what you're holding onto. How are you breathing? Dreaming? How do you react to things? Your body reflects what you're thinking and feeling. It's brilliant and should be trusted totally!

I was looking to my body for information about what to do and how to let go. I could tell by how I felt in my body if I was doing the right thing, because I felt good. If I felt uncomfortable, I'd notice and shift what I was doing. I paid attention. Getting my health back was more important than anything else, so I concentrated on listening both physically and emotionally. For the first time in my life, I could finally take a deep breath, slow down, and concentrate on me.

Getting quiet and centered is a big part of listening to your body. There's no way you can listen well to what your body has to say unless you are truly focused and silent. You absolutely need time to reflect, to open up, and to feel your own presence in a peaceful setting. This is nurturing for your body and heart and settles your mind. You give this to yourself — the time, the space, and the energy to focus on your insides. Direct your mind to your body and focus on all of it bit by bit, being attentive as you move from head to toe.

Think less about what's happening and see if you can feel more. You don't need to think about anything while you're in your serene space, reflecting lightly on how your heart is beating and how you're feeling. Gently touch your heart and remain there and feel gratitude well up in you. Be completely relaxed as you think the thought, "This is all I need to do. I am paying attention to what I'm feeling for myself and this body. This is my only purpose right now."

Letting go of hard feelings will help your body let go and regroup. Every day have some quiet time to reaffirm your commitment to releasing pain, judgment, or resentment, and replace all of it with gentleness and peace. This is a gift to your body. You can look in the mirror and decide to be the one who heals yourself. You are the one who decides, from the minute you wake up until you close your eyes to go to sleep, how to use the power of your mind in each moment. Use your quiet time to help your body heal. Gentleness and patience affect everything around you, and expressing that brings a healing energy.

Don't be afraid to use your intuition when deciding how you can care for your body — what to eat, when to rest or exercise, and what to do when you're feeling sick. Trust what comes to you suggesting what you should do. Overrule what your head says you "should" do. Have faith that your body knows everything it needs, and all you have to do is listen. Your body is a constant reflection of your mind, so it will tell you when things are out of order.

Monitor your thoughts as much as possible. Being attentive to what you're thinking about is a practice and takes patience. Little, passing thoughts that you have all day when corrected can change the way your body functions. Loving, healing thoughts and being grateful are the most powerful ways to improve your health.

You cannot fool your body.

It understands your mind on the deepest levels. It's the information that you continually feed your body that makes an impact. One time, random thoughts that are not accepted mean nothing. Thoughts that you find yourself saying over and over again will affect your health and well-being. What you believe will have the greatest influence on your health. You have unlimited potential for health when you practice positive thinking.

Be aware of what you listen to and what you concentrate on.

Your mind is highly influenced, especially when you're told you're sick. Know that your mind is the best tool you have to help your body get better. Don't fill your mind with negative advice and statistics. If you want to do research about an illness or injury, just remember that any information you're looking for can be found on the computer. That means anything — if you want to prove something, you can — from both sides. Don't believe all you read.

In a recent article in the *Wall Street Journal,* "Why Placebos Work Wonders," Shirley S. Wang explains how the mind-body connection is changing the way doctors look at patient's response to drugs and information during illness. She writes, "A particular mind-set or belief about one's body or health may lead to improvements in disease symptoms as well as changes in appetite, brain chemicals and even vision, several recent studies have found, highlighting how fundamentally the mind and body are connected."

If a sugar pill (placebo) can change the way you respond to an illness, imagine what a doctor's opinion can do. What if a doctor has an opinion about your case that is just not true? It could possibly create a situation where you believe something that changes the outcome of your illness in a negative way. What you believe is what's important. Not all doctors are as good at verbal healing as they are with medicines and procedures. And sometimes they are absolutely wrong.

Interesting story: When I had gone through my double mastectomy and gotten the results of the pathology, I was told I was a stage 4. This is a pretty big deal – I was shaken by the number. It was then put into my chart and a permanent part of my patient folder. It was only a number, but it made a difference to how I felt. There was never any question as to whether it was true or not and it became a part of my journey.

Three years down the road, I'm in an oncologist's office in Phoenix, Arizona. I have just moved to Sedona and I need a doctor to prescribe my ongoing drug treatment (10 years is protocol for my type of cancer). I find a very good cancer center and have my records sent from Rhode Island. I meet the doctor, have the exam and get my prescription. When I go to say good-bye, the doctor mentions that my file has me as a stage 4. He says to me, "I've looked over your records twice and you're a 2B".

All this time I've been thinking and believing that I'm something that I'm not. It didn't matter that it wasn't true because in my head, I knew what the doctors had told me. So I didn't know that I wasn't a stage 4. For all intents and purposes, I was a stage 4 for three years. If you believe it to be true, that's what it is. I have a few tattoos on my forearm and one of them says "Accept it as truth and it is yours."

What you don't know doesn't matter.

Ignorance is bliss. There's a lot to be said for that. Going your own route – following what you believe and being aware of what you think is important to staying centered and healthy. If you're in a program with a doctor, you can still concentrate on what's important to you and ignore everything else. Turn off the news, stay away from negativity in relationships and information, pay attention to what you think is good and true, and believe that you're well.

– 11 –
A Meditation for Healing

Y our body is a massively complicated organism working twenty-four hours a day, every day, just for your well-being. Approximately 150 trillion cells are reacting every second to keep you healthy, comfortable, growing, and thriving. At this moment, your body is crazily busy regulating your temperature, digesting your food, taking air into your lungs for your blood, beating you heart 100,000 times a day, getting rid of toxins and assimilating nutrients, filtering your blood to form urine, and on and on. And we don't even notice it! We forget that there is a whole universe of things going on to keep us alive. We take for granted that we'll take another breath, and we don't have to keep track of any of it.

The body's job is to take care of the package that holds who you really are — your spirit. This package is constantly changing in relationship to its environment. By taking time to create an environment of growth, you help your body to heal. Looking at the marvel of our bodies is not something that we often do — and hardly ever with gratitude. Try to imagine this meditation as a thank-you response to your body. No matter what situation you're in right now, a thank-you is always appropriate.

Sit comfortably and close your eyes. Relax and take some deep breaths. The aim right now is to be as relaxed as you can possibly be. Go into your body by bringing your thoughts to what's going on with you right now. You might have an ache or pain. Maybe you're a little hungry or thirsty. Unclench your jaw and relax your eyebrows. Open your mouth a little bit, and let your tongue soften. Let your shoulders relax; breathe deeply. Feel your hands — those amazing appendages that help create our daily lives. Feel the energy in your hands — the buzzing energy — and appreciate it.

Move on to other places and appreciate them. Rub your feet and toes long enough to let them know and feel your attention. How great does that feel? They hold you up all day! They are amazing. Your body thrives on this attention and affection. Feel the energy in your belly and put your hands there, showing your love. Remember where your rear end is? That wonderful place that we feel comfortable sitting on (sometimes for too long) that doesn't get much credit? Give thanks for what's behind you. Appreciate the neck that holds your head up all day — move your head in a circle, slowly feeling all the creaks and cracks. Roll your head around until it feels more fluid. Give attention to those areas that are stiffer than others. With your hands, grab the upper part of your back below your neck and massage it while you roll your neck. Feel the body responding to your touch — it loves your touch and caring.

Think of your insides — all the trillions of cells working for you. Thank them and be grateful for them — send them your loving energy. Be totally relaxed while appreciating your inner workings. Feel a tremendous gratitude flow through you. Smile a little. Sit with it while you remember to relax your mouth and forehead and breathe deeply. This is the feeling that your body is looking for to be at its best — to be in the growth cycle. When the body is relaxed and feeling safe and loved, it responds with contentedness, and then it can concentrate on whatever it needs to do. Being relaxed and feeling the flow of your body is when the body has time for repair.

Feel your body healing. Know that it is what it wants to do — it's trying to heal all the time whether you realize it or not. Give it the chance to heal free from stress and fear. Know that your body is a natural healer, and that's what it's doing now. When you feel the love and gratitude for your body, it responds with growth. The longer you can stay in this state, the better. You have no stress, no worry, and no fear — only feelings of gratitude. Feel completely relaxed, safe, and loving, and know that your body is responding in amazing ways. Know it, believe it, and trust in it.

– 12 –
Stress on the Body

I knew I was carrying things that put stress on my body — sadness, resentment, unfulfilled dreams and desires. Keeping track of my painful memories took a lot out of me. Our bodies are not meant to carry heavy emotional loads, and when we do, it shows. The regret and resentment that I held put a huge drain on my body and took all my natural energy. I never realized how much of a drain they were on me until I started letting go. Coming to terms with guilt, resentment, sadness, and any hard, heavy feelings will immediately improve your health.

Any painful experiences that you hold onto in your body can be damaging. Whether it happened yesterday or thirty years ago, if you haven't dealt with it, it's causing some form of stress. You know the memories I'm talking about. We've all had them, the life-changing ones and the little, hurtful ones you can't forget. You have to let them go.

When you get serious about letting resentments go, I found that journaling about them really put the memory in perspective. When I wrote it down, I wrote it from as many perspectives as I could. Knowing what people are dealing with at the time of a crisis is impossible. This in and of itself brought me healing. Knowing that we all do our best with what we're given made it easier to forgive. Also, now that I am much older, I knew that things happen differently than you want them to even with the best intentions.

I let go of anything I could think of. The big memories came first. I wrote everything down that I could remember, and then I would write down why it still hurt and how I wish it had happened differently – looking at it from different angles. I tried to examine why I thought it was worth holding all these years, and why I couldn't let it go until now. Every single time I went through this, I felt a shift. Some of the memories I wrote about several times before I could feel forgiveness.

Stress on the body is what causes illness. Is holding onto memories long gone worth making your body sick? Really? Think about this. If you could forgive someone and relieve your body of the drag it's causing, wouldn't you do that just to feel better, to feel lighter and free? Not to mention letting the other person off the hook feels fantastic. I want to be healthy, not stressed. I did the forgiving for me.

– 13 –
Nurturing

When I found out I had cancer, I took care of myself better than I ever had in my life. I nurtured me like I'd never done before. The attention that I gave to my body and my emotional needs was first and foremost on my list for the day. Nothing was out of the question. If I needed something to make me comfortable, there was no guilt getting it or doing it. For the first time in my life, I became worth it — what I needed, I provided for myself, and I never felt any hesitation at taking the time and attention to stay comfortable and relaxed.

This is when you have permission to take nurturing yourself to a new level. Whatever you need, do it or get it — now is the time. A nap, a special book, a walk, going early to bed, a cup of tea, a friend, a heating pad, a new pillow (or three) — find what you need and give it to yourself. Spoil yourself, and if you can take off from work — do it. *Do not underestimate your job.* Your job is to take such good care of your body and your thinking that you can heal and begin to thrive again.

The attitude you assume when you nurture is that of love. There is no way to nurture and not be caring and gentle. So many of us don't feel enough love for ourselves to be able to nurture well. We have spent the last half of our lives taking care of our families and friends, and we just aren't used to paying attention to ourselves.

The act of nurturing doesn't have to be an appointment or scheduled event. You can just take a few minutes out of your day to do what you'd like to do. A nice walk, a twenty-minute nap, or taking time to read an article you've been holding onto. If you are intent on nurturing during that time, you will be. The focus is on you being treated well. The definition of nurture is the care and attention given to someone or something that is growing or developing. You are always developing and growing — day in and day out. Take time for yourself to feel the care and attention only you can bestow on yourself.

Where you put your focus is the key. Focus your attention on giving what you need to yourself. Attention is the best form of nurturing. Give yourself permission to rest, relax, read, and enjoy whatever it is that would fill you up. Ask yourself, "What do I need?" When you start to realize how deserving you are of your own affection, it'll change the way you look at spending your free time.

– 14 –
Moving

What I've learned about moving my body is not what I've read or learned at the gym. I've learned it by doing, and then seeing how I felt. It's not conventional. Kind of like everything else, I did some listening to my body, and it told me to move certain ways. I might have been motivated to move more because of all the surgeries I'd just had. After a double mastectomy, all the radiation that tightens your skin, and then a colon resection, I really needed rehab, but I wasn't up for generic gym work.

I needed a way to release tensions in my body. I did some breath work in a workshop, and while I was heavily and purposely breathing and listening to music, I cried and cried. This caught my attention. I was curious about what I was holding onto, and it made me wonder what I had buried deep down inside.

The only way to release these buried energies was to move and breathe in ways that would let them go. I knew that by breathing hard and very deeply during the breath work, I'd touched on some very big emotions probably from way in the past, but who knows? When I started thinking about these emotions being trapped in me and wanting to come out, I wondered how I could do that and get cleared of any pain I might be holding onto.

I've been active my whole life, but in a very predictable way. When I was a kid, I did a lot of bike riding, walking, swimming, and group sports. As I got older, I began doing more routine things like power walking, lifting weights, a little running, some elliptical at the gym, but mostly the same stuff.

Think about how you move.

It's usually so predictable. How does your body get rid of energy trapped inside if you move the same way all the time? It gets stuck. Now you might think I'm crazy, but I tried some different things and got some very good results.

First of all, we underestimate the lack of real movement we actually do. Like everything else in life, we get used to moving a certain way, doing things in a certain style, and getting into a rut. I felt that breaking out of that rut was important.

It all began by doing back bends in the shower. Yes, I did. I had this sense that I should be bending backwards. I went with it. I had a wall right behind me, and I would balance my hands on the wall behind me while I bent backward. I did this every day and made my way down, tile by tile, one day and then week at a time until I could do a backbend outside on the ground. I considered the energy that must have been trapped and released in that back bend — in my chest, hips, upper arms, and upper back. When is the last time I'd done a back bend? I think in seventh grade.

This is why yoga has such a huge following — the breathing, the stretching, and the moving. The problem for me was I'm not really a yoga person. I know that yoga would do the same kinds of things for me that I ended up doing, but it's not something I was drawn to. I made up my own stretching by determining what my body told me to do to release.

I began at the gym doing things that I hadn't done before. My body wanted to be pushed, I could tell. The first thing that I noticed was the more I sweated, the less hot flashes I got. How come nobody ever told me that? As a matter of fact, they completely stopped. Also, the more I sweated, the better my metabolism was, and I started seeing much better results in my muscles. This made me really happy after all the surgeries. I got excited to go to see how much more I could do. My energy level was increasing, and I knew that my body wanted more.

Do we assume that because we're not trained athletes, we're just going to be older women that move a little slower and a little less? I know I did. I stopped really pushing myself once I hit my late 40's. My body wasn't convinced that was the right move...I began to see my body as something that could still grow and learn and be better.

I would stretch in ways that seemed very natural for me — just kind of feeling it out. Letting my body tell me where I needed to stretch. If you put yourself in a position and keep moving and stretching until it feels right, then push it a little more. That's what I did more and more each week. I got a routine going. I did "my" stretches for twelve counts each and did them while breathing deeply. At first, I did this in a meditative state. The whole stretching segment would last ten to fifteen minutes, and then I'd meditate.

I purposely focused on releasing energy. These positions are not what we learn to do — they're for my body, and they feel right for me. I think everybody has stretches that are specific to that body. We all move differently, and we all need to stretch to suit the individual muscles we use and especially don't use.

At a certain point, I started stretching to music, which led me to dancing. When I say dancing, I mean what you would do if you were absolutely sure that you were the best dancer on the planet, and nobody could see you moving to your favorite song. The rhythm from music helps you to move in ways you wouldn't normally do. I can't begin to tell you the energy that I've released doing this. Not to mention listening to great music, letting off steam, burning calories, being as limber as I've ever been, and feeling so happy to do it that I can't wait for that part of the day.

As I aged, I'd stopped stretching my body and pushing it's limits. I think this was natural, but a mistake. We tend to slow down as we age, but at least for me, I could see that the decision to do that was from my mind, not my body. My body is in no way ready to slow down. Of course, I have a few more aches and pains, but far, far less now that I'm back in shape. The pain comes from slowing down, getting stiff and out of shape. Once you realize that you are as in shape as what you do, you can regain some confidence in your physical abilities. The only way to get your body up and running again is through movement. Never underestimate a really good sweat. The more you stretch and move, the better your body will function. No doubt about it.

I exercised every day during my treatments. Even in the dead of winter, I bundled up in a warm coat and hat, put the dog's leash in the car and off we'd go. Every day we went - fresh air, moving my body as best I could and appreciating the ability to be outside.

One last thing about exercise. I believe that our bodies need to breathe lots of fresh air and be outside as much as possible. Take in the beauty of the sky, feel your feet on the earth, and experience our Mother. In order to stay healthy, our bodies need sunshine, deep breathing (oxygenation of the blood), stretching, and moving in ways that keep us young and lithe. Spending time outside in a garden, at the beach, in the woods, or mountains is not just good for your body, it's what your soul wants. The more time you spend outside, the better. Working out at the gym is great, but it's not the only way to get in shape, and it certainly doesn't feed the inner you.

– 15 –
Higher Guidance

What if you could improve your overall health by changing your mind? What if you decided to look at situations from a different viewpoint and your body responded with terrific health? There is some very new and cutting-edge research being done on the influence your point of view has on your health and well-being. Imagine that what you perceive in your surroundings is actually effecting how your body functions. When you believe that things are good, your body acts in a way that promotes your health. And when you're worried, your body prepares for disaster, neglecting your growth and focusing on your protection.

Your mind and body work together to help create the life you're living. Your body takes care of the package that's you to the best of its ability, and your mind spends most of its time thinking of things that are of no use to you whatsoever. Sorry, did you think you were making better use of your time? Your mind thinks approximately 60,000 thoughts a day. It is estimated that 98 percent of those thoughts are literally the same ones you had yesterday, and they can be geared to the negative and mundane — that's the way the ego wants it.

How can we get our minds to help us instead of hinder us? Controlling your thoughts to live a more healthy existence is all about focus and attention. Focusing on the positive will give you positive results, and the opposite of that is also true. If you can get your thoughts to be positive and uplifting, you'll have that kind of life. It's really that simple, but you have to monitor what you think. Perception is where you choose your experience. If you choose to perceive your life as a positive experience, it will be. That's it. Letting your mind run the show leaves your ego in charge, and it's not going to let you believe that life is good without a struggle.

Jill Bolte Taylor, a Harvard-trained brain scientist, had a stroke and realized very clearly which side of the brain she was thinking with. She wrote a book called *My Stroke of Insight* to help stroke victims recover and understand what happened inside the body. Her discoveries were special in that she explained what was happening to her from a personal as well as a clinical perspective.

She wrote, "My anger response, for example, is a programmed response that can be set off automatically. Once triggered, the chemical released by my brain surges through my body and I have a physiological experience. Within 90 seconds from the initial trigger, the chemical component of my anger has completely dissipated from my blood and my automatic response is over. If, however, I remain angry after those 90 seconds have passed, then it is because I have *chosen* to let that circuit continue to run. Moment by moment, I make the choice to either hook into my neurocircuitry or move back into the present moment, allowing that reaction to melt away as fleeting physiology."

"Neuroscientific research indicates that experience can actually change both the brain's physical structure (anatomy) and functional organization (physiology). Neuroscientists are currently engaged in a reconciliation of critical period studies demonstrating the immutability of the brain after development with the more recent research showing how the brain can, and does, change."

All this means is that science is changing the view of how the brain works. What science believed before, that the brain did it's developing in early childhood, has completely been challenged and is now no longer regarded as true. What is believed now is that your brain's ability to develop new neural pathways, changing the way the brain functions, can be brought on by new experiences — environmental and behavioral. Literally, just thinking different thoughts will change your chemistry and in turn change how you feel and who you are. Did you know that smiling changes your body chemistry and boosts your immune system?

You might believe that who you are reflects your personality, but that isn't really so. Your personality is composed of repeated behaviors that have been happening since you were conceived. These behaviors were based on how you responded to situations. You cried when you were hurt, laughed when things were funny, and felt loved when you were hugged. The relationships that you've had in your life have created situations that you've responded to again and again. These responses can be viewed as your personality type. Certain personalities act in certain ways. Personalities, however, are not something you are; they are ways that you've acted and can change at any time, if and when you want.

All feelings have a chemical makeup as your cells respond to experience. Joe Dispenza explains, "What you think is what you experience, and when it comes to your health, that's made possible by the amazing pharmacopeia that you have within your body that automatically and exquisitely aligns with your thoughts." In his book *You Are the Placebo*, he explains how your thinking creates the chemicals that make what you believe possible. Our brains make what we think and feel come into reality by chemically creating what our cells need in order to create change.

Your body is also capable of making chemicals that mimic the drugs you might take to recover from an illness. You have to believe you can recover, and then the body makes it happen. If we expect to recover, the body responds to that expectation. Our brains don't know the difference between taking a medication and taking a placebo — it's the expectation to get better that makes us better.

With this in mind, consider what you think about on a daily basis. If you're thinking negative thoughts all day — day in, day out — your body is creating chemicals that keep you awash in negativity. This reality that you're perpetuating for yourself will have physical effects that can change your health. You don't realize how effectively you can make your body sick when your thoughts are chronically subjecting you to chemicals that reflect your negativity. You can see that by underestimating the power of your thoughts, your body can be directly affected by a daily barrage of your mind's negativity. The only way to counter that is by changing your thoughts to positive ones.

For instance, the experience of feeling angry effects your body's chemistry as do all emotions. Feeling angry has a certain chemical response, and if you analyze the experience in your body, you can feel your body react. For anger, your heart might race, your face may get red, you might feel tightness in your chest, or hold your breath in — this is all in response to your body's chemical change, not just your emotions.

Every time you think a thought, you create a chemical. The chemicals are called neurotransmitters. Your cells respond to what you're thinking, and they react a certain way. When you think the same thought many times, the neurotransmitters create a new neural link from cell to cell, creating a pathway. The more you think the thought, the stronger the path. This is what happens when you learn something new. A new pathway is formed, and you can retrieve that information again as something you learned.

Your thoughts create feelings, and when thought again and again, they create a familiar feeling. Your body gets used to feeling a certain way. In the body, this is chemically recognized. When we develop a familiar feeling, it becomes comfortable. Even if the feeling isn't comfortable in situational terms, like getting angry at someone, if you're angry enough of the time, the body feels a certain level of comfort because it's not new.

Your body and mind work together when expressing emotion. The mind perceives an event, and the body follows with a chemical reaction, which then reaffirms the mind's perception. When someone does something that you sense is an attack; you react with angry words. When you react, the physical symptoms kick in brought on by the chemicals created, and the body shows the mind that it's angry with the sensations of anger — so now the mind and the body are on the same wavelength with actions and feelings used together.

As you get older, feelings that you experience continuously become your natural ways of reacting. We call that your personality. Your responses become familiar to your body as well, the chemical reaction, so much so that your body misses the reaction when you change your behavior. This is why changing what you do normally (considered your personality) to something new can be very uncomfortable. You don't feel like "yourself." The only thing that makes you feel better initially is to have the same behavior, so you go back to doing things the way you did before.

Your body actually tells your mind what it thinks it's missing from the chemical standpoint. Then your mind tries to get you to reestablish your old, familiar way, telling you, "This new way isn't working. Look how tired and hungry you are. You need a bowl of ice cream," or whatever the old pattern was. The body will work on getting the mind to do what it wants to get that feeling — even if it's bad for you. This kind of back and forth between the body and the mind doesn't really have anything to do with what's good for you or what's in your best interest or even your personality.

What's wrong with this picture? None of this is happening with your involvement. It's all just triggered responses. You are being run by the body/mind, and unless you turn that whole process inside out, you won't have much of a chance of changing your behavior. You are totally out of the loop. The ego and the body are running your life, and you are acting in ways all day long because of a dialog between them.

Getting off the merry-go-round so you can actually change a behavior is difficult, because it's not easy to be in touch with why you do things on a moment-by-moment basis. Once you've become aware of the "why" of all of this, it should be much easier to access your higher Self and find a better way to act. When you really want to get to a place of change, you have to be able to make sense of the "why," so you can observe what you're doing and start to put the new way of acting into play.

The mind is what brings the experience to the body. Through the senses, the mind perceives what's happening in the environment and in turn tells your body what's going on. It doesn't even have to be true, and, in fact, many times it's not true. Have you ever watched a really scary movie and had your heart race, throat tighten, and eyes closed, and then you hide behind a pillow? That wasn't happening in reality, but your body didn't know that. In other words, it never has to be the truth to affect you. It can be anything you perceive and believe.

The body's senses see, hear, and feel what's happening, the mind interprets that based on past experience, and the body creates physical feelings to go with it. So, in a sense, you are at the mercy of your body's reactions to past experience, unless you examine the situation and reassess. Past experience might not be at all applicable right now. It might even be detrimental to you at this moment. In order to live on a level of awareness that keeps you healthy and in the present, you must consider your actions and how you participate in your relationships going forward, not from what's happened in the past.

If you get angry, your natural tendency, or your "personality," might normally yell to defend yourself. In order to effect change, you decide to do what is new for you, and it's not going to be comfortable. That doesn't mean you can't stay with the uncomfortable feelings and learn to react in a new way. You can say to yourself, *Wait, I don't want to do this anymore — I'm going to try acting differently.* You relax and breathe and notice a feeling of calm, and then work with that.

Learning that your body's "voice" tells your mind that it's feeling abnormal goes a long way to help cope with the unnatural feelings you might have when you want to change a behavior. Your mind, by itself, also has an agenda. The ego will chime in whenever it feels it needs to assert itself to be better, smarter, or stronger. This is why we learn not to believe our thoughts when they're not in our best interests.

Learning new ways to behave in old, familiar situations can be one of the best ways to create health and wellness. First, it makes sense to find the behaviors that are not serving you well. Getting angry, frustrated, or impatient stresses the body and chemically triggers the fight response. The way to calm the mind and the body is to get quiet. Whether you're with people or by yourself, you can get to a quiet place in your mind and choose to be peaceful. If you don't feel peace, something's not right.

Going deeper into your body then where you are normally relaxes you and helps you listen. Looking at your thoughts and emotions when you're reacting to a situation is where you start to learn about yourself and begin to question why you act the way you do. It's not your personality per se; it's your learned behavior. And it's not permanent or unchangeable.

One of most effective ways I learned to change what I used to do is to not react at all. Take a time out. Walk away and don't say a thing until you can act with purpose. Defending myself is the easiest way to fall back into old behavior, but I've learned that by not responding right away, I can think of something funny to lighten up my natural response. I can admit to being exactly what I was accused of and go even further by making fun of myself. This undoes my old feelings of vulnerability. It makes me feel powerful not to defend — the opposite of what used to happen to me. Instead of separating myself with defense, I join in the relationship with humor.

– 16 –
A Healthy Point of View

A sk yourself honestly what you believe about your health, or if you are ill, your illness. Listen to the answers. If it's not positive, you can change the way you think. In changing the way you phrase your thoughts, you can alter what you think to be true. It's not as easy as just saying it once or twice. In order to really change how you feel, and what you believe, it takes commitment and perseverance.

Watching your thoughts and getting to the truth of what you believe is an ongoing practice. It is not something you can do in a day or a week. Catching negative thoughts is a very effective way to help improve your health. Practicing every day to monitor your thoughts and develop a more positive attitude and gratitude for your body and your life could be better than any medicine.

Make a choice every day to be as healthy as you can possibly be.

Physical and mental efforts go together and can't work without each other. You can't think wonderful, healthy thoughts while lying on the couch watching TV all day and expect to stay healthy. You also can exercise and eat well and have negative thoughts ruin all that you've been trying to do. The balance between your thoughts, beliefs, and your physical surroundings is what your life is made of. Choosing health deliberately — inner and outer — takes motivation and effort, but when is a better time than now to be motivated?

– 17 –
Getting Quiet

T he more often you can train your mind to get quiet, the faster you can feel the benefits. You can notice quiet anytime. Getting quiet and spending a little time alone every day, whether you officially "meditate" or not, is important. Meditation is very personal, and there are many ways to make it work for you. You can start with ten to fifteen minutes at a time. If you can't do it every day, then just try to fit it in when you can — in the car, while waiting for a doctor, before you get out of bed. In other words, it's better to get quiet more with less intensity than not at all.

There's a part of your mind where you can find stillness. I have a place in my head where I can hear the wind and see a sky. When I go there, it helps my body recognize that I'm going to meditate. My body gets ready to quiet down. Once I have settled on the sky and the wind, I can shift into a quiet place. Sit comfortably in a chair; you don't have to sit on the ground and assume lotus position to make it count. Sit or lay down, it doesn't matter, and it depends on how deep you want to go. If you're interested in a thirty-minute, really intense, deep, and completely quiet moment, then close the door, sit, and turn your phone off. Meditation isn't about being perfect — it's about touching on a quiet place in your mind.

I believe it's very beneficial to just sit and get very relaxed both in body and mind. The change in your energy is what you're looking for — the chance to totally calm down and rest in the moment. Getting still is very healthy for your head and your body. Many people won't meditate, because they're afraid they're doing it wrong. There is no wrong. Don't worry about it, just do it. Get quiet and pay attention to your breathing, that's the easiest. You can say a word over and over again. You can watch thoughts come and go. You can try clearing your mind gently every time you find a thought arise. It really isn't about doing it right or wrong. The point is to do it enough that you start to feel comfortable and you feel your mind shift from busyness to a sweet, soft quiet. Once again, this is about what's right for you, what makes sense to you.

Just walking quietly outside and purposefully calming your thoughts is a wonderful way to get quiet and have clarity. Thinking while you're walking, going over questions you have, or analyzing your responses while taking one step and then the other is very beneficial and clearing. It's a little like meditating with your eyes open. Call it walking meditation.

What you want to do is to consciously stay calm and open to what comes up in your head, but then let it go. No looping. A thought that just keeps coming back again and again in a loop is more like obsessing than meditating. Ask questions and wait for answers. Look at the answers and wait for more — quietly and calmly examine what you hear in your head. Don't have an agenda. This way of looking at what's in your head is very calming and can be really productive. I always finish a walk like this with positive thoughts to my questions.

Meditating can drastically reduce the time it takes to analyze your own stuff. You can see how that would work. When you're busy interacting, you're not aware enough of your motivations for acting the way you do. Calming the mind and choosing to find the truth in what's going on in your head will come quickly using meditation. Changing your behaviors can only come when you recognize what it is that you're doing, and more importantly the "why."

– 18 –
Mirror Meditation

Here's a great exercise in seeing your higher Self. Go find a big mirror and stand right in front of it — close enough to see into your eyes. Stand there and really look. Relax. Look into your eyes and see past your face to your Self. Stay there and keep looking. You will find that you can see past your body, past your little self, and into the eyes of your higher Self. You might feel a little uncomfortable, because you can absolutely tell you're looking at more than your body's eyes.

She's in there. There's a timeless wisdom there behind those eyes. The body is her house, and the mind helps her/your body get along in this world. She's watching your whole life happen. She's your Inner Eye. She's there watching you, experiencing through you and loving you. She has compassion for your pain and for your happiness, but she feels none of it on the body level. You are how she experiences this existence.

If you look long enough, you can look right at her. They aren't just your eyes anymore. You have to do it long enough to make your face not matter. The structure of your body is irrelevant. What you look like doesn't mean anything. The exercise is about seeing past your body into the infinite wisdom contained there. Your higher Self is here to experience through your body and mind and observe. If you wait for your body to drop away from what you see, you'll feel an intense connection to something more than who you call yourself.

This exercise gives you a glimpse of how much more you are than a body. Your body is what you think is you, but it's just a little fragile piece of what "you" represent. The body is merely an idea that gets you from point A to B. It's a way one Soul can experience another here on Earth. Don't get carried away with your body and mind. They are tools to be used by you so your Self can learn and grow. Remember how much bigger you are than your body, and it will put things in your life into perspective.

– 19 –
Manifesting Health

W hen I realized that it was me who needed to change in order to get healthy again, I had to figure out what I was doing wrong. I've come to a lot of understanding looking at the way I act from the perspective of an ego self and a higher Self. When I analyze what I'm doing and feeling, I always try to find the motivation behind it. The simple way of seeing how I operate in my mind and body gives me a great vantage point for awareness and change. The way it makes sense to me and how I can work through change is by breaking it down into simple pieces. What I call myself when I refer to my ego is my "self" with a small "s," and when I'm living through my heart with wisdom, compassion, gentleness, and intuition, my "Self" is with a capital "S."

Jill Bolte Taylor breaks it down to the two hemispheres of the brain. In *A Stroke of Insight,* she says that the ego, small self, is the left hemisphere, and the authentic self is the right hemisphere. "Many of us speak about how our head (left hemisphere) is telling us to do one thing while our heart (right hemisphere) is telling us to do the exact opposite."

A Course in Miracles says that the two parts of your mind are the ego, which represents fear, versus the Holy Spirit, which represents love.

So whether you believe it's the left and right side of the brain, the little self versus the big Self, or the ego versus the Holy Spirit, it doesn't matter as long as you know you have a choice between the two.

I believe it's possible to change if we want to — to change what we think, what we believe, and who we are. I don't believe anything is permanent. Your personality and genetic makeup are just pieces of the whole, and with the right information and viewpoint, they can be changed. I think with the right way of looking at what you do, you can understand and then practice a new way of behaving. I'm not saying it'll be easy, but it's possible to live anyway you choose and be anybody you want.

Your higher Self is the part of you that knows what to do regardless of what you've done before. It can override the body and the mind and help you find new ways of doing things. Your higher Self can hear the body and the mind, but it cannot be ruled by it. This is when you start to realize that your reactions are not you. There is another part of you that can see and feel what you're doing and just observe. You are so much more than the body and the mind — those are merely your instruments in this life. They're ways of experiencing life as we know it, but it's not you. Your higher Self can also be called the Inner Eye, because it merely observes.

Your Self can assess a situation and make a call that isn't always in line with what you think is your best interest. For instance, letting someone win an argument. Your ego will always put up a fight with your higher Self. Part of you might want to stay and argue, but when your Self steps in, you immediately know, because you have a sense of peace and calm. There's no mistaking a decision made by your Self versus your self. The ego just wants to be right, to be safe, to be the best and smartest; your higher Self wants peace for everyone. The ego doesn't care about the fall out; all it cares about is defending its story and protecting what you look like at face value. Your Self is willing to let the story go and be vulnerable, because it knows there's nothing that can really harm you. This brings a true feeling of peace, and peace makes you happy and healthy.

Your higher Self can be reached anytime by being calm and quiet. There's too much going on with the body and mind to figure things out while you're in the middle of doing and reacting. The best way to get in touch with your Inner Eye is with quietness. Ask yourself questions and you'll get answers. This is what I call higher guidance. When you feel peaceful, you know you're on the right track, and when you lose your sense of peace, you immediately know you've chosen the wrong part of your mind to make a decision.

Your higher Self has the power to set anything straight by understanding that what your mind is telling you isn't true. Get used to the idea that it's a combination of chemicals and past experiences that are leading you to do what you do. If you don't like some of the things you're doing, change them. It's so helpful to understand what's really happening to you on the inside, and that can give you the power to shift.

The mind-body connection is completely underrated. I believe that your thoughts can change your body. I believe that what happens in your head is directly reflected in your body. This is the reason for all my searching and learning, and I'm hoping to change how I thought and viewed the world. I want to think healthy thoughts, so my body will reflect that and become the proof that it can be done.

You can't bury your beliefs, and you can't override your body. When you think you've overcome something — a feeling of resentment, a feeling of betrayal, or even a very stressful event — the body's reaction is what will tell you what's true. You might think you've recovered or forgiven, but you really need to observe your reactions to see the truth. When you feel pain or lack of peace, you know you still have work to do.

The way to find out what's in your subconscious is by observing how you act in your relationships.

When you feel your peace disappear, you're reacting to what you believe. This is a good thing! Losing sight of peace is what lets you know you've got buried stuff. It's not enough to say you've forgiven someone or even think of it — you need to know you have, or your body will hold it and try to heal, but it won't be able to. How you react in your relationships is the only way to get to know how you really feel, not how you think you feel.

Healthy thoughts are not just about what you're eating and doing; it's a way of looking at your life. It's a certain direction that you turn when you are faced with a "problem." It's knowing that everything is fine, no matter what happens. Letting go and feeling peaceful and positive is healthy. Staying in a loving frame of mind is healthy. Knowing that there is goodness all around you is healthy. Knowing that you don't have to do anything to prove your worth is healthy. Loving yourself and nurturing yourself is healthy.

Let the body do its job taking care of you by understanding why it does what it does. Figuring out what reactions you have that DON'T serve you — holding onto old behaviors that are damaging and feeling emotions that seem out of control — will aid you in getting your health back and also help you understand what needs to be changed. Try to remember that the body and the ego have an agenda, but they don't have to rule you. You always have a choice in how you act and what you believe.

What will it take to change what you've been doing for many years? How will you act the way you want instead of jumping to the old behavior? If your higher Self is where all your wisdom is, then how do you get there when it really counts?

All it takes is to understand what is happening on your inside. It's all about awareness. If you can notice what you're doing and understand why, you can change it. The answer is that once you understand that your mind and your body are stuck in a habit of reacting to certain situations, you start to do something different or you're going to be immersed in the same old behavior. Doing something different is a choice. You just choose to act another way.

First of all, swallow your pride and admit you've got some behaviors you don't want. Admit it to the people who will be affected, too. Remember, this is learned from years of experience and mind-body reactions. Don't blame yourself; everybody's got their stuff. Just work on changing. Don't try to defend yourself. Start by trying to understand what it is you're doing and reason your way through it. When I stopped defending and started trying to be loving, it changed me dramatically. It made it so much easier to say, "Yah, you're right. Can you believe I did that? Wow, what was that about?"

Your body reacts to your feelings, and those feelings can create an overall chemistry to your system. Years of acting the same way kept me in a climate of negativity. I was always worried, resentful, and guilty. There was no part of my day that I reflected with gratitude. There were very few times that I totally relaxed and enjoyed what I had. I was busy and focused on things that didn't matter, which in turn was reflected in my chemistry.

Bruce Lipton, a genetic scientist, wrote *The Biology of Belief*. He studies epigenetics, which are changes in gene activity that are not caused by changes in DNA. In other words, those are the changes in an organism outside of DNA. He believes that your thoughts dictate how healthy you are. How you perceive your environment is what tells your genes how to respond. Your genes actually can't predict much until the cells receive information from the brain about the environment. Our cells respond to different perceptions of our environment.

There is growing evidence that will change the way we look at our bodies going forward. For the last fifty years, science has believed that our genetics were the determining factor behind how our bodies responded. Although the fact that you have brown eyes and hair are strictly controlled by your genes, your development and ongoing growth is controlled by your perceptions and how you feel about your life. This means that cells respond to what you think.

Your environment and your lifestyle dictate your tendency to stay healthy or to create disease. Healthy lifestyles, good clean nutrition, exercise, and a happy, positive outlook in life keep your cells in a "growth cycle." The growth response from the brain promotes health and well-being. It takes care of your organs and your general health. When you feel stressed or threatened in any way, the protection response puts you in survival mode, which ignores your general well-being, putting all the body's energy into a ready-to-fight state.

If we feel safe and happy, our cells work towards growth and repair. When you perceive a loving and positive environment, you are relaxed, and your body only sees the need for growth. If you perceive your surroundings to be hostile and negative, your body responds in a certain way — to protect you. If we feel threatened, our cells will spend their energy preparing for defense. Do you perceive your environment as loving or hostile?

Only one can happen at a time — either growth (no fear) or protection (fear). Your belief about the life you are experiencing determines the way your genes perform. Are you stressed at work? Are you worried about your health, money, marriage or your kids? Think about how much you worry. Worrying is fear, and that creates a situation where you feel threatened which works against your general health.

There are only two choices you have in any given situation. You can choose love or you can feel fear. One choice is going to be good for your body, and one is going to put you on the edge. There is nothing in between; everything comes down to those two things. Everything. Our egos are set up to keep us fearing everything — all things, people, events, time — you name it. That's why you choose not to believe your thoughts. That's the ego talking — and the ego has a BIG agenda.

All the time you spend worrying is time in protection mode. There's no room for growth and repair there. If you worry a lot, you never give your body a chance to be in the growth cycle. No repairs are being made, and constant stress is put on your body. Your body cannot stay healthy without the growth cycle. Lighten up and enjoy. Stop worrying and feel the positive vibes of relaxation, appreciation, gratitude, and happiness. Your body will then begin to heal, and it's only during these times it can heal.

As we grow and develop, chemical reactions activate and deactivate parts of our genomes. These chemical reactions are influenced by our surroundings and our perceptions. A genome is all the information of an organism's heredity. Your heredity plays only a part in your health. Your perceptions control your biology. Your biological information is not determined solely by your genetics, and, in fact, may be an extension of your environment — what you're exposed to, what you do, and what you believe. Your genetic code that you were born with was thought to be absolute, and you were powerless over the traits that you inherited. This left you a victim of your genes. Scientific evidence now proves this is not the case.

How your body changes and grows is not so much driven by your genetic makeup as by how you perceive your environment. This means that you can't blame what's going on with your body on your genetics. Your genetics have very little to do with your health. You have a great deal of power and control over how your body expresses the genes you were given. Your perception and your point of view are going to alter your body's course more than anything. It's possible that your thoughts have a bigger impact on your health and environment than that of physical matter. So controlling your thoughts could feasibly be all you need to control your health.

– 20 –
Habits

A nalyzing the reasons why you respond to a certain situation in the way that you do is the best way to get to the bottom of the whole behavior.

For example, when I come home from a long day, the first thing I do is get something to eat. It doesn't matter if I'm hungry or not. So why do I do this? When I was younger, I lived in a household that was stressful, and food was a comforter for me. I was often nervous coming home, wondering if I was walking into a bad situation. I know that when I come home now, nothing will have changed. I live alone, so there's nothing there to be afraid of. I can now look at my craving for something to eat (even if I'm not hungry) as a habit that doesn't serve me anymore.

If what you're doing isn't healthy, or it sabotages what you've been trying to do, then making a change makes sense. Why do you act in ways that don't serve you? Because of habit. Looking at the habit and the whys of the habit will shine a light on it that helps to break the pattern.

I didn't know I wasn't focused before the cancer. I thought I was focused on my life, my work, and my kids. But I wasn't. I was distracted. I was keeping busy with things that didn't matter. There was always that relentless sense that if I wasn't busy doing anything, I was slacking. If I was slacking, then I wasn't worth anything. Pretty simple philosophy. My life was on auto-pilot and run by my habits.

I thought I had a purpose, but it was just many different things all bundled together — no focus. I was letting life unfold without being present — kind of just catching up when the next thing came. I let my day be directed by what I'd always done before. My habits actually caused me pain, but I didn't even know it until I really looked at what I was doing.

When I got cancer, I found my focus. With this new found focus and the time I had to spend on learning, I went about changing a lot in my life. There was a lot that wasn't working for me currently. I wanted to hit the reset button. Habits are only good if they reaffirm what you're working towards, like a healthy lifestyle, a loving attitude, or a dedicated time to learn.

What you choose to do should contribute to all your goals — that's where the focus comes in. I thought I was acting the way I wanted to, but I hadn't looked at what I'd been doing for years. I hadn't analyzed any of my behavior to see if it was what I really wanted. What I was habitually doing did not contribute to what I wanted to achieve.

Once I realized I had habits that were directly opposed to what I really wanted, I had to change them.

In this sense, I worked on being a grown-up more than anything else. Children want what they want when they want it, disregarding all the consequences. That's why children are not left in charge of what they need and want — they have those choices made for them.

As an adult, we make much better choices for our children than we do for ourselves. We can and often do forget that we have responsibilities to ourselves and our bodies. We want something and we get it — we eat it, we drink it, we do it — *"hey, we're grown-ups; we can have it if we want it!"* If we were acting responsibly, we'd choose to do something different a lot of the time. If we had to make the same choice for someone else, like our children whom we loved and cared about, we'd say "no."

Just because you are able to put something in your mouth doesn't mean you should. Just because you can watch TV for hours every night doesn't mean you should. Just because you can drink the whole bottle, doesn't mean you should. You must act like a parent to the voice in your head that wants what it wants and will try to convince you to do it. It is important to recognize the demands of the child within us and to be enough of an adult to make wise choices.

Now that I'm aware it was my chemistry that was perpetuating a lot of my habits, it was easier to change them. Doing something different for thirty days starts a new neural pattern. Continue to do it for another thirty days and you're firmly implanted with a new habit.

Being a grown-up means making choices that might not be so popular with your inner child. Understanding what is right for you because of experience and personal knowledge is easy if you're in the right frame of mind. The higher Self will make choices based on fact and not on want. To realize that what you want is not necessarily what you need is putting your higher Self in charge. You don't act on every want, but you assess your needs and decide when to fulfill them. It sounds like very little fun but actually, it's where happiness comes from. I'm not talking about being a stern, strict grown-up, just one that has your best interest at heart.

Being happy has nothing to do with getting what you want.

In Laurel Mellin's books, *The Pathway* and *The Solution,* she uses her system to help control how you behave. One way to look at being a grown-up is confronting the "essential pain" of not getting what you want and the "earned reward" of feeling good at the end of the day, having accomplished what you set out to do.

It has to do with an inner balance and being able to count on yourself. Happiness does not come because you wanted a doughnut and you ate it. Think about it. You might be excited eating the first bite, and it might have tasted good, but after it's eaten, are you happy? Nope. That's not happiness. Happiness comes all through the day, when you make choices and decisions that are good for you. The respect for yourself makes you happy. Feeling good about your decisions makes you happy.

We get so wrapped up in the habits we used to cope with. Time goes by, and before you know it, a habit becomes a part of your character. If someone were to call you on it — what you've become — you might even deny it, because you've been denying it to yourself all along. How does the jump to cover hurt feelings, anxiety, fear, and restlessness become a habit; become such a big part of you, that you don't remember how to do it another way?

Day in and day out you reach for something to ease your pain — a cookie, a drink, a pill to sleep, whatever it is. It becomes the way you cope. Coping day to day without facing those feelings — ignoring them and reaching for a substitute every time you're uncomfortable — will eventually change your character. A little here, a little there, and in time it's a part of you.

Remind yourself who you want to be. Maybe write down who you thought you were and see if you're still there. For me, I realized that I had gotten bitter, resentful, and hard-hearted. That's not who I thought I was, but it was how I was habitually acting. I thought I was really healthy, but I was eating when I wasn't hungry, drinking wine every night, and zoning out on the couch. Ouch. Not who I wanted to be. Habits got me there. Little by little, I became someone that didn't reflect who I thought I was.

– 21 –
Zoning Out

After having a close call with cancer, I don't waste much time, or, if I'm being really truthful, I just don't. I don't even own a TV because I have so much else I can do that I love. I feel strongly that if I'm living an authentic life, I can do anything I want, but it won't be about getting away from my life — it will be about enriching it and engaging in it.

I used to spend a lot of time "resting" after work, and what that really meant was zoning out. I numbed myself. I did not nurture, which is different. Nurturing is about taking care of what you need to grow and learn. It's not about numbing. If you need time to rest, then rest and you can still do things that are beneficial to you, but not zoning out. Reading, hobbies, dates with friends, meditating, exercising, or caring for your body — you could be busy for the rest of your life taking care of you.

I am not saying that escaping doesn't have its place — but know that you're escaping. Also, I am not talking about having fun. Fun is nurturing. Being with friends and hanging out watching TV is different than the ritual I created. Getting in the habit of having a drink and watching TV for three hours every night is wasting three hours every night. TV doesn't give much. There is nothing in that for you. Write a book, learn a new skill, volunteer your time, make something, develop yourself — put time into yourself, nurture yourself. Love yourself.

When your ego senses that you're trying to break old habits, beware. You are up against the trickiest form of bullshit on the planet. Your ego knows exactly what will get you, what makes sense to you, and it will manipulate you perfectly. Watch your every move and never underestimate the conniving story the ego will tell you to get you to return to your old ways.

Old ways are safe and support the ego's story of you.

Brace yourself while you remember that your ego is not in charge. Your habits are not something that need support, but examination. Your higher Self needs to be available all the time when you're breaking a habit. It takes a lot of searching and examining to get past your story to the truth. The truth is that you don't need to listen to the ego — and when you get this you are free.

When you're trying to change behavior, you might want to give yourself extra time to do things — periods of quiet, reflection, and rest to let your Self check out what is happening. When I'm busy, I realize that I am not really paying the kind of attention it takes to act in my best interests. You need time to notice how you feel and to analyze what's going on in your body.

In Scott Kiloby's book, *Natural Rest for Addiction,* he talks about resting in the present to get past cravings. "By noticing a craving energy in the body and letting it come and go without emphasizing any thoughts about it, the craving loses its capacity to fuel obsessive thoughts." You need to be ready, though, because your mind and body are working in tandem to get you to go to the same response you've always had.

If you're only moving on old energy, out of habit, the chance that you'll be able to change behavior is not likely. Whereas, if you have time to yourself, you know you'll be able to breathe deeply and relax and look at how the day is going. You can sit with the present moment and see where you stand. You can see what you could do to calm down and focus, and you might actually be able to get to where you're doing what you'd like to be doing. Habits take great energy to break. If you really want to change, you'll need to challenge that energy with an equal energy.

Destructive habits will begin to fall away when you begin to love yourself more than you want to escape. Here are some habits that disappear with love:

1. Treating your body badly
2. Wasting time
3. Avoiding contact
4. Negative and critical thoughts
5. Talking about other people with judgment
6. Procrastinating

– 22 –
Habits Become Character

Sometimes it takes crashing to change. A full-blown, head-on crash to see where we were. Seeing what kind of person our habits have made of us can be shocking and may not fit in with the view we hold of ourselves at all. Our view of ourselves can be what we hope we are — what we strive for. The problem is that denial will lead you to believe that's what you really are until that crash. Cancer was the way I crashed.

Once I was shocked into seeing myself, it was devastating to see how far off the mark I'd travelled from what I wanted to be. And I had such good intentions! Then I started to understand why the crash happened — why the event, the diagnosis, happened in the first place, and I was grateful. I never would have woken up — I was thinking I was pretty close to who I wanted to be, but I wasn't. It was crushing to be so disappointed, but that helped with the energy I needed to change.

I was jumping all the time to get away from myself. My habits came from trying to escape myself (it's pretty hard to do) — my restlessness, boredom, and anxiety. I forgot who I was and who I ultimately wanted to be. The crash brought me back. It was a gift. I crashed into myself, my habits, and my actions when I got cancer, and I saw myself clearly for the first time in many years.

There's an endless repetition of behavior that makes us ask, "Am I crazy? Why am I doing this again?" And until you reach that new level of understanding about yourself, there's very little chance you're going to see where you really are. Keep the compassion and the love coming, because the only chance of pulling out of your chronic destructive tendencies is kindness. That's the only way. Beating yourself up just causes more of the same stuff. Kindness and nurturing will help you grow out from under unwanted behaviors.

Your internal voice, the self, is not an authority, although it'll sound like it. It's quite the opposite, and it's not always wise. Your higher Self needs to kick in and help with the choices you make. You can use your Inner Eye as an internal monitor to keep you on track and happy about your choices. The Inner Eye needs calm and quiet to stay in touch, so if you plan a little time for noticing what you're feeling and doing, it'll be easier.

With more peace in your life and more reflection, your body responds by telling you whether what you're doing feels good or not. The motivation for giving up what your body doesn't want is the knowledge that with the space you create by giving things up, you are leaving space for other more important things to come into your life. One door closes and another opens. You leave space for the unknown path to show itself — it doesn't matter whether this is in regard to your health, your relationships, or habits.

It still won't be easy to change your habits, because you've got the body-mind working to keep the status quo. With the knowledge of the "why" and the understanding of the reasons you started acting that way, you can open that door to the possibility for true change. As Michael A. Singer says in *The Untethered Soul,* "If you really want to see why you do things, then don't do them and see what happens."

The bottom line is if you feel uncomfortable, check your intentions. You'll be able to see the ego at work, making things complicated and twisting the truth to suit its needs. Quickly observe what you're doing, so you don't get too caught up to turn around.

– 23 –
Your Story

"It is possible to move through the drama of our lives without believing so earnestly in the character we play."

— Pema Chodron

My story is what I believe to be true about my life in its entirety. My history explains my story. I have a story in my head about who I am — we all know the story of ourselves. When we believe our story to be all of who we are, we play into it. We do things that make what we believe real. We are identified with what we think we are. We hold onto the picture of what we think our story is so tightly that what happens plays right into what we believe. What we believe to a large extent is what will happen. Your story unfolds as you believe the story will. When you lose the story, it changes everything.

"I'm here to be me, which is taking a great deal longer than I had hoped."

— Ann Lamont

Without a story, you open up to possibilities.

Being open to what might happen and keeping your story as just an idea, instead of identifying with it, brings new things into your life. Your life is on a path, and whether you direct that path to align with your story or not is up to you. In order to let go of your story, you have to believe that you're not defined by your history or what you've perceived as your history. This takes a little waking up to do.

You need to interrupt the momentum of your existence long enough to see how swept up in the whole picture you are. What we call our story and being so identified with it makes it hard to picture ourselves without it. Who would we be if we let it go? To just be. Just be who we are right now without anything to back it up. Imagine walking into a room full of people who don't know you and not telling them your story — no background. You'd have to be okay just "being" who you are at the moment.

Imagine not filling your day with what you know how to do. What would you do if you didn't have to prove who you are? I know for me this is a huge test of whether I've given up believing my story. If I can't let you know what I've done and where I've been, what I'm capable of, then I lose my agenda. If I'm not concentrating on impressing you and proving things to you, then I can pay attention to you. Wow, what a concept.

When I started talking about what was going on with the cancer, something inside me didn't feel right

— I wasn't sure what was different, but I was having a hard time telling the story of my cancer. I'd gone through things that were sad, scary, and seemingly unlucky, but that was before I felt sure I needed to look at my way of explaining my life differently. The old story got stuck in my throat. My life and the way that I looked at my life seemed too dramatic. I didn't need any more drama. I wanted to look at this event with a new definition of myself.

When everything started to shift for me, the story telling did, too. I would begin to explain to someone about what had happened, and the drama would dissolve – it just started fading away. The truth was enough. I realized that looking like the victim of the events of my life had no appeal anymore. I was not going to act like a victim, because I knew I was ready to take responsibility. I didn't feel the need to change anything that was happening right now. It all seemed to be enough and just so, without any extra anything.

When I got cancer, I had to look at everything I was doing again and again. I felt it was my job — my life was on the line. Eventually, I got to most of what was causing me pain, but it took more than a year of soul searching and honesty. I realized that I was acting out a victim story in almost every aspect of my life.

I never thought about how I put a spin on things. I never noticed that if I was telling a story, I would give it a flavor to make me look a certain way. This is how we keep all our events fitting together to continue the story. The spin is what makes the story fit more securely into our identity. This was so powerful when I first noticed it, the story of me and how I'd done such and such. I put in the little extra words to embellish my story — the slight shift in focus to make it fit what I thought was more "me" — as though the plain facts were never quite right.

The reason for the drama when you got right down to it was that I didn't think I was enough without a good story. I started to see myself telling stories over the years about me and what had happened to me and the drama I wanted to create. Most of the stories actually are pretty good without any spin at all, but I still felt as though I had to change my tone to look more like a victim.

The problem with spin is that it tells yourself things that you begin to believe. If I was always spinning a story to make myself out to look like I'd gotten the raw end of the deal or the victim of an accident or was unlucky — then I was those things. This becomes your truth. I didn't want that! What was I thinking?

I was not going to be a victim any longer of anything. I'd started taking responsibility for what was happening in my life on every front, and I no longer wanted to tell a story that wasn't totally true, and in fact, I wanted it to be uplifting and inspiring. I also no longer felt the need to do it. How do you want to appear to others? Is there an underlying spin to your experiences when you talk about them?

My story started taking a backseat to what was happening right now. I began to lose the desire to prove who I was by providing the details of my past. I was no longer so busy trying to make you see who I was trying to be. There's a lot of energy there — in the proof. The challenge was talking about my new situation without the back story. Let's just talk about the facts. I knew this was healthy. I thought that my life depended on it. Looking at myself as a victim was not going to help me through the illness, and I didn't need to "make" this part of a sad story.

The story that I'd been telling for fifty years was one of hardship at a young age, divorce, death, alcoholism, and not enough love or nurturing — lots and lots of us have a similar story. What I considered my misfortune colored everything I did, because I believed it was what made me "me." I carried it with me and loved to revisit it, because it validated everything I'd ever done. I had reasons and excuses for my behavior. I didn't have to take responsibility for the things that had happened to me, especially at a young age, and I felt justified and competent for doing so well, given my situation. I was fulfilling the role of myself in the play that was my life, and I was very wrapped up in it.

– 24 –
Pain Gives Way to Peace

As I considered my story, I saw a lot of patterns and thought processes that became eventualities. When I started to realize that everything that had ever happened to me was a direct or indirect result of situations I had created myself, it was life-altering and painful! In one moment, I was a woman who had had a lot of incredible events that "happened," and, in the next, I had created them all. Holy cow, that kind of realization will stop you in your tracks. That shift, to a certain extent, saved my life and began a change that would turn me completely around.

Waking up requires a commitment. It is so easy to slip back into old behaviors — especially defending yourself! Defending our own story is a full-time job for some of us. You absolutely need to question your view of why things have happened the way they did. When you find yourself putting together the pieces of why you did certain things, check to see what kind of story they're telling. "Well, I did that because she said this, and then I decided that it would be better to go there because..." Do these things fit into a story that you're already telling?

The story is only a story that nobody but you is following closely. Nobody else cares about your story; they've got their own to deal with. You stream together all your experiences to make you who you think you are. You are so much more than your story and much less, too. You limit yourself by your story.

My story of being the victim of unfortunate events was something I secretly loved. I wouldn't ever have called my life unfortunate, but I did have experiences that made the story viable. When I was diagnosed with cancer, I could have continued the drama if I wanted to be a victim — getting cancer fit right into the story of victimhood. Imagine that! Actually, it was so perfect that I knew it had to be the next big thing that I'd created to keep the story going. Isn't the ultimate victim a dying cancer patient?

At this point, when I started to get it, that it was me playing a role and creating a disease to continue being a victim, I was so shocked I couldn't completely believe it. It's actually pretty easy to do — just concentrate on something day in, and day out for years and it'll happen. Think of your story this way: What is it that you want in your life? If you want it, you can make it happen. But even if you don't want it, by concentrating on it, you make it happen. The Universe does not distinguish between what you want and what you don't want — it merely provides what you concentrate on. It's a very simple concept.

Going through life thinking that you're doing your best and bad things keep happening to you is a way to avoid responsibility for your actions. If you feel you don't have a choice as to what you experience, you'll never take responsibility. We are never a victim, but not realizing that, we can spend years defending our victimhood. There are people who don't want to own what they do. That's okay. There is no rule that you have to follow. If you're not ready to take it on, then don't. However, if you want to take charge of your life, if you're sick of having no control over what seems to keep "happening" to you, then facing your actions and their consequences is the only way.

I completely owned my cancer. I was ready to leave being a victim behind. I couldn't even get the old story going; it just died in my throat. It never occurred to me to feel sorry for myself or be a victim — cancer was too serious for me. The truth in my story woke me up. I needed to stop doing what I'd been doing, or maybe not live through it. I instinctively knew that playing the victim role created weakness. This was not a time to be weak, and I knew that. Survival takes power and strength, great faith, and the belief that you can change what is happening in your body.

You must believe that you'll recover.

You put recovery into your story. You must hold onto your strength. The truth is that you absolutely can turn your health around — by yourself. The ONLY power you need to recover is your power to change your mind. Changing your mind — one day at a time — can save your life and bring you back to wellness and health.

I took responsibility for my illness. Whatever was going to happen to me was going to be my choice. I knew that I had created what was going on with my health, and I knew that I could create a new story that I'd be happy with. The situation I was in was a culmination of many events, but they were MY events. I knew that I had brought this all to me — not only did I know it, but I understood all the whys. If I created it, then it was possible to change it, and I was determined to undo what I'd done. There was never a doubt in my mind that I could fix what had gotten out of sync in my life. I knew it was up to me to change what I'd become.

I believed that I could change my health with my thinking. I was new to this realization. It still made sense to me to continue my treatments and surgeries, along with my new way of thinking. I was far enough along with my cancer that I wasn't sure I was strong enough or had enough time to turn my health around without medical help. I am content with the choices I made, but I think, going forward, I would put a lot more faith into what I can accomplish with my thinking.

You can go to a doctor — get all the necessary help and treatment, surgeries and chemicals — but if you don't clear up the things that helped to get you into the situation, you will probably wind up right back where you were. A body can't hold onto all the things that made it sick without responding in the same way. For me, it wouldn't be breasts again, because I'd lost them. But there would be another illness if the thinking behind it didn't get cleared up.

I needed to clean up my act — clean house, so to speak — get in all the dark places I'd ignored for so long and start being truthful about how I'd been acting. I somehow knew this. It wasn't something I knew before, and I didn't learn it. I just knew it was the truth. I listened to my Self. I understood that I had to change my ways. By looking at the story I'd been telling, I could tell what had to happen to change it. I had to forgive a lot. I had to let go a lot. I had to start allowing and stop judging, controlling, and manipulating every situation.

Unresolved issues: painful memories, betrayals, resentments, and feelings of being wronged are all feelings with stories behind them that yearn to be resolved. Holding onto the hurts of the past is damaging to bodies — we know this — you can feel it. It is painful, and anything painful can be faced head on and repaired with time and forgiveness. We all have very distinct and separate histories. We are completely individual and so are the ways we will heal. What I needed to do was just for me and what someone else will need reflects their unique past.

When something — actually anything at all — is painful, it is calling out for attention both physically and emotionally. That's why there is pain. Emotional pain and physical pain are there to call attention to whatever is happening that isn't right. It's a survival mechanism, and we all so often avoid it or deny it — shove it away. When something hurts your body or your heart, pay attention to it and figure out why and what is going on.

– 25 –
Are You a Victim?

It's possible that taking the role of "victim" could hurt your recovery. Not everyone is able to take responsibility for their illness, but it's the mind-set that makes a difference. What you've thought about and what you've done, on the whole, have played a part in what is happening in your body and your world. You have played a role in what happened, but that doesn't mean we're talking about fault at all here. It's about awareness regarding your thoughts and actions, not blaming yourself. Recognizing what your role is or was can change your life and save it, too.

Unwrapping myself from the victim role wasn't that hard really — it just took awareness. I'd been acting like a victim since I could remember, and seeing my "story" as that of a victim helped me to change much quicker. Once I saw what I was always doing and saying, it stopped. It's not that difficult to see where you are in your story; change your outlook — your position. Ask yourself how you define your life. If you had to explain it, would it be happy, satisfied, or grateful?

When you look at who you are portraying to people around you, it can become obvious how you would describe your story. What you assume about yourself will be reflected in your past and how you act now. If you aren't well, it's important to see how you define the path you've been on. Illness says a lot. What you believe about yourself will be played out one way or another, and if you want it to be a "good" story, you've got to figure out what you're saying to yourself and to other people.

When your story isn't serving you or doesn't feel right, it's the perfect time to shift gears and take on a new definition of yourself. In my case, when I talked about cancer, I switched from a victim position to one of positivity and strength. Any negativity I was tempted to express literally stopped before it formed into a full sentence. I have continued with this to the best of my ability regardless of what I'm talking about. Energy is attracted to similar energy. I don't need negativity in my life.

It's all in your viewpoint. It's how you approach your actions. What you do in conjunction with your intent is what creates the energy. For instance, if you believe that doing things for others will get you what you want, you're doing things for the wrong reasons. That good energy of doing something for someone else gets combined with getting what you want, and that creates its own energy. Your acts of kindness are not going to keep you from getting into trouble if your heart's not in the right place. The intent wasn't genuine so the energy is off. If you believe that you'll get the short end of the stick, you will, because that's viewpoint/energy, too. It's what you believe and what you concentrate on that will manifest itself and perpetuate your story.

It's very hard to help yourself if you feel everything is everyone else's fault. How can you help yourself when you think the control is in someone else's hands? No amount of talking and support will be able to get through to you unless you can get past who's to blame and understand what's happening underneath. There is no one to blame. To honestly answer the question, "Why me?" is better because it'll open up more of what's going on. Ultimately, there's just you and its no one else's fault. Question your attitude more than anything in form. Make the whole picture of your life into an overall sense of attitude and see if that's what you want for your future. Is the general feeling of your life positive?

When you drop your story, your mind is free and at peace — it is not conflicted. When your mind isn't conflicted, it holds itself open and vulnerable. It's not trying to prove anything all the time. It's learned to embrace and accept the truth about the mind itself — which is to observe what you're thinking, but not believe it. It is willing to be truthful and to cultivate a deeper honesty with what's happening right now.

There's no longer any pretense when you stop trying to make the story work — there doesn't need to be — because you're okay with what is. You're not trying to appease the ego and be better than someone else. There is no story to uphold. There's no longer any effort to control and manipulate how you appear or worry about what people think of you. There is no unconscious energy running the show. The mind is relaxed and transparent to itself — it feels easy just being here. There is no hidden agenda, and therefore you feel at peace. This is a practice and I continually come back to check on where I am – am I trying to uphold a story or am I just being who I am right now?

> "If it's never our fault, we can't take responsibility for it. If we can't take responsibility for it, we'll always be its victim."
> — Richard Bach

The ego wants to be right. We make the ego feel good when it's someone else's fault. We can spend lots and lots of energy trying to appear innocent and right. Our ego feels strong when it gives the responsibility for our problems to something other than ourselves — this can only leave us as the victim. But being a victim steals your strength, and you need your strength, especially when you're not well. You want to keep your strength and the belief in your own ability to get better. If you stay responsible, you keep your strength. Don't give your muscle away. Own your experiences and love them for making you who you are.

If you choose to be a victim, then you are choosing to let life take you on a ride where you have no control over where you're going. You have chosen to be swept away with anything and everything that comes into your path. It probably won't be all bad, but there's a chance that maybe it will. It's all a guess when it's someone else's fault. Victims are at the mercy of any and all events that come their way.

Being a victim implies that something happened to you without your participation. Although no one would ever consciously choose to get cancer, there are definitely things that you can do to help bring it on. Owning the fact that you might have contributed to your illness makes you responsible, and believe it or not, this gives you power. Figuring out exactly how you might have contributed to your illness gives you even more power. With that knowledge, you can begin to make changes.

Even if you don't believe that you've played a part in your illness, there is always room for change and self-exploration. When you take charge of your health while being proactive and staying positive, anything is possible, and believing this can change your life. There is ancient wisdom in you. Don't deny it — believe in it. Putting energy into your recovery can give your sense of involvement a lot more power, and it will have a healthy impact. You can hold yourself up and be responsible for your part in what is happening to you right now or let events take you for a ride.

> "As long as you think the cause of your problem is 'out there' — as long as you think that anyone or anything is responsible for your suffering — the situation is hopeless. It means that you are forever in the role of victim; that you're suffering in paradise."
>
> — Byron Katie

You can ask yourself questions to figure out where your thoughts are coming from. "What is it I'm after?" "What's my motivation?" "What do I really want?" "How do I want people to see me?" "What is the lesson here?" "What part am I playing?" "Where is my heart in this?" "What kind of thinking brought me to this?"

The right question can break through hours of wondering why you're experiencing this right now.

Questions are the easiest way to get the answers, and I need answers to understand the part I'm playing. My life is full of experiences that have been brought about by certain patterns in my thinking. These patterns were largely unknown to me until I started asking questions. I want to have an idea of what I'm doing subconsciously — what I'm creating.

> "Every person, all the events of your life are there because you have drawn them there. What you choose to do with them is up to you."
>
> — Richard Bach

You're control lies only in what you think and how you respond.

Everything in the Universe is part of a gigantic play of creation. You have no control over the play, just how you participate in it. When you are faced with the possibility of your life ending, you see quickly what matters and what is unimportant. I finally understood that I had control over how I would participate in this life and how I would make it all be on purpose. I would transcend my circumstance and my story and realize the opportunity I had here, because this IS a serious opportunity. Every minute is an opportunity to choose how you want your life to unfold. It's totally up to you.

> "The decision to overlook the seeming inequities of life instead of reacting to them is a choice."
> — David R. Hawkins, MD, PhD

– 26 –
Power versus Pity

F eeling like a victim can leave you feeling weak, and you don't want that, especially if you're sick. Feeling weak when you have an illness can increase your sense of vulnerability. You need your energy to feel healthy. You may not be sure that you have the ability to correct what's going on in your body, but that's okay if you remember to keep a positive, strong attitude. If you feel out of control and at the mercy of your illness, there is a much longer way to go to get better.

Feeling pitiful comes from a place of inadequacy. If you feel inadequate to face what you're up against, it'll be harder to recover and get better. Feeling inadequate is a story you're telling yourself. It's an opinion that you're choosing to believe. When you feel responsible and powerful, you'll believe you can change what's going on. You have to believe you are MORE than adequate and have the capacity to help yourself.

It's not a healthy energy to feel sorry for yourself, and I prayed that I never would. I prayed for mental strength. I tried to be proactive most of the time to keep from feeling scared or weak. I believed in my doctors, my treatments, and my full recovery. I believed it, and so I lived that way. I lived as though everything was going according to plan, and I would be completely healthy in no time. Every blood test, every surgery, chemo, etc., was in perfect order, and even if I got some news that was not wanted, I'd get over it as quickly as I could. Do the best with what you've got today. No stories about being a victim — no stories, period.

Pity feeds victim thinking. Pity makes you feel and act weak. I was very careful about being with anyone who felt pity for me. I'm really sensitive to pity and could feel my energy shift dramatically when someone was feeling sorry for me. I stayed away from people who showed their caring through pity. Showing compassion is great, but feeling badly that someone is sick is not helpful. Being loving, giving, and caring is helpful. Feeling sorry for me didn't make me feel that you loved me more, and certainly didn't make me feel any better physically.

> "Asking for pity is believing that you are weak. Suffering is increased and multiplied by pity. Pity spreads suffering."
>
> — Aristotle

People who are dealing with an illness do not need you to feel sorry for them.

Not at all. They need you to love them, that's it. Help is wonderful and appreciated — help with meals, rides, cleaning, support — whatever you can do to help is great. Your attitude as a helper is immeasurably important if you want to create a strengthening atmosphere. Pitying someone who's sick will create sadness, weakness, and victim thinking, which is not what you want to create. The best way to give someone strength is to love them and make them feel worth that love.

I learned a lot about how to be a good caregiver from my mother-in-law. She was a tremendous support. She was there for most of my chemo and surgeries. She gave me exactly the kind of care that was right for me. There was never any pity. I was very happy to have her there, particularly, because of her attitude. Attitude is THE most important factor when dealing with anyone's illness. My mother-in-law gave me great advice on many occasions, but during this particular time, what she told me changed the way I might have handled the whole experience. She said, "Get up every morning, put on your clothes, put on your makeup, and make your bed. If you have to get back into bed, that's okay, but start your day like you always do." I was filled with purpose and strength following that advice. I acted like it was any other day.

Jill Bolte Taylor wrote some things that she needed for a full recovery of a stroke in her book *My Stroke of Insight*. The following are some that pertain to all illness and I completely agree: "I desperately needed people to treat me as though I would recover completely. I needed those around me to be encouraging. I needed people to come close and not be afraid of me. I needed my visitors to bring me their positive energy."

As a caregiver, it's more important to be positive and strong than anything else. As someone who's ill, it's not always possible to be positive. I am not saying that you shouldn't lose control and grieve for your situation. Sometimes it's better to let loose and get it out. I am not saying it isn't awful to have cancer, or to love someone with it, to be afraid of dying and to feel pain.

What I'm saying is that telling yourself a story about your cancer and making it into a tale of "woe is me," feeling sorry for yourself, and allowing people to pity you is not the way to get better. That's all I'm saying. If you're interested in recovering fully, feeling healthy, and learning from the experience, then being part of a sad story is not where you want to be.

You are responsible for your thoughts and your actions, and both of those things will shape your present situation. Thinking like a victim and getting people to agree with you only enforces the fact that you are out of control — by choice. My son and I call it victim venting. Its a little game we play: you're allowed to do it if it doesn't go on too long, and also that you realize you're acting like a victim. You can complain, blame, justify, and then you let it go.

We surround ourselves with people who will agree with us — rallying the troops to get lots of pity and go on and on with the story. This is what friends do, right? I don't think so. I think agreeing with a victim story just keeps it going when nothing gets accomplished by it. Have compassion and understanding, but you don't necessarily have to agree. I got to a point where I didn't have time to listen to that anymore. Complaining gets to be just a waste of time for the complainer and the listener.

> "Embrace your heartache and love your struggles. This is your life."
> — Pema Chodron

Even if your body is weak, your mind can be full of strength. Feeling like a victim and accepting pity will only keep your disease in the forefront. The idea is to keep the body thinking like a healthy body, not to continue to tell the body it's sick. To treat your disease, you must get past the illness itself to the core truths that played a part in getting sick in the first place. Believing in your total wellness is the best place to get your body and mind working together for your ultimate well-being. No matter what you feel like physically, you can keep your mind strong and feel gratitude for the moment you're in.

– 27 –
Changing my Story

U p until this time of change, I'd been a black or white kinda girl. I had an absolute opinion on everything. Even if I didn't know, I thought I did. Now that I had cancer, the grey started to settle over all those opinions. Had I been wrong about everything? I decided that the answer was pretty much a "yes". It was a bit freeing to feel so wrong. What the hell? Starting over wouldn't be so complicated if I questioned everything I'd thought was true. It was an opportunity to undo all the beliefs that I'd been holding onto.

I was happy to start over. I felt a wave of strength in certain areas — the ability to grow and change was exciting. I never questioned why I got cancer. I never said, "Why me?" I wasn't good at being a victim now that I saw it clearly, and this was life-saving. All that being sure of myself with strong opinions and judgments just dissolved. Some of the strength backing up that behavior helped me find the courage to admit how wrong I'd been. It's much easier being unsure than it is being sure. Being sure takes a whole lot of energy to back it up. Being unsure, I could float.

It was almost as though I had been waiting my whole life to shift my perspective. I had been so "right" that I couldn't bear to change what I thought and how I acted without a real reason. Here was a great reason. It felt like a door opened, and I was just waiting to go through it. It was inviting me. It was the idea that I'd been thinking things were absolutely the way they were, and then all of a sudden there was no truth to it.

I had been waiting for the moment that was so tremendously important that I'd have permission to change everything I'd been doing. When the moment came, it was cancer that gave me the ability to go through that door into uncertainty. I stopped living the way I'd been living. I just stopped. It was time to shift my entire perspective. After all, what I'd been doing got me into this mess — it was time to make some radical changes.

Looking to myself for the reasons that I got cancer has been the most enlightening, uplifting, and positive experience of my life. I'm talking about reasons that give me a basis to begin again from scratch. I'm not talking about who to blame here. There is no one and nothing to blame for anything, and I mean that. Blame doesn't solve any problems, and it makes no sense to waste time and energy on blame.

Blaming is also more victim behavior. Blaming your mother, your father, your childhood, your husband, job, the government, whatever — it doesn't matter when you know it's really all about you. It's not about anyone else. Pointing a finger will not help you and certainly can't fix the problem. Blame is a way to pass the responsibility to something or someone else, which, of course, is possible but not helpful.

What I'm talking about is being responsible for what I can control. Being able to change all the things I can to live a healthier, more balanced life with lots of joy and gratitude. I wanted a reason to continue on in my life that wasn't attached to my ego's story of who I'd thought I was. I wanted to be free of my past resentments, regrets, and pain, which were all part of the same thing. I wanted to feel responsible for my happiness. I wanted to know what it felt like to be full of love and peace — to be free of the play I'd been acting in for fifty years.

So, coming to terms with my part in all of this led me to take a different road than the one I had been on. Even though I had to admit how misguided I'd been, the emotional pain wasn't that bad with all the new potential I saw in front of me. To get to know myself, I would have to take down the walls that I'd put up in defense of my own pain and look at all of me. Taking down the walls was only a matter of believing that I could handle the pain and open up to it. Feeling the pain, whenever it came, got to the core of it. All I really did was acknowledge that I was in pain when I was. Facing how I felt and my resentments was uncomfortable after so many years of avoiding them, and I came up against a lot of resistance. But I was willing, and sometimes that's enough.

My story contained a whole list of things I was capable of doing. I was capable in many areas, and this defined me. I "did" them all day long. I spent years of my life doing things to prove that I was valuable. I finally realized that my story about doing and being perfect wasn't going to make me happy, nourished, or fulfilled. I kept doing and doing, and all it made me feel was tired and resentful.

I missed the point to everything because I was busy! I needed to "be" more to survive. I was doing so hard that I couldn't see what was happening — waking up and just making more lists. I found out by getting sick that my "doing" wasn't enough to sustain my soul, my authentic self. I thought I was living an authentic life, but it was the picture of the life I wasn't really in. I couldn't see who I was and what I'd become.

The moment came, thank God, when my body showed me that I needed to look at what I was doing and shift gears — or die. I knew the minute I slowed down enough to stop the doing, and it only took a week or two — that I was so off course. This had to be the reason I was sick. I was waiting for the whole show to collapse before I could slow down enough to look at what my story had become. In hindsight, it seemed so obvious, but I didn't see where I was going because I was so consumed. There was no time to reflect and I think that was why I had stayed that busy. It was a way to escape

To change my story I simplified. I became slower. I became more present and aware of what I said and did. I focused. I took a lot of deep, thoughtful breaths. I concentrated on what was important. I did what I wanted to do. I cared more about the little things that I kept in my life. I engaged more with people and forgot about all the "shoulds" I used to have. I stopped trying to prove myself through what I knew how to do and just started paying attention to the people in my life. And one of the biggest turn arounds came when I began to play.

– 28 –
Stress Memory

During my cancer year, I was plagued with intestinal problems. Anyone who's been on chemo drugs knows how hard it is on your body. I had been chronically dealing with colon issues for close to forty years, and it was so bad during chemo that I had to seek more help than just a gastroenterologist.

By the time I was forty-nine, I had been diagnosed with diverticulitis twice (infection in the colon). I was so used to the pain that it was a fact of my life, but it had gotten so much worse in the last few years. I thought that being diagnosed with cancer was a much bigger deal, but, as it turned out, the colon trouble ended up being a huge issue. It was very difficult to get my mind off the pain and discomfort in my lower belly and at the same time try to deal with the cancer treatments and surgeries.

Not one gastroenterologist ever could help me, and believe me, I went to many. I had six colonoscopies between the age of thirty-five and fifty years, and none of them helped diagnose the problem. I had at least three doctors trying to help me during the time of my breast cancer. It was suggested that I have surgery to remove the part of my colon that was getting infected and not working right, but it would have to wait until my cancer treatments were over. Nobody suggested another option.

So when the majority of my treatments were done, I decided to try some alternative therapy for my colon. Kerstin Zettmar was recommended to me by a friend of mine, and what she taught me was life-changing. She uses the Rosen Method, which facilitates touch and words to explore the subconscious root causes of chronic tensions in the body. Marion Rosen (1914–2012) was a pioneer in treating psychosomatic illnesses. She focused on the mind-body connection and emotional stresses.

Kerstin and I talked all through our sessions, and, while we talked, she touched me and massaged my body. She worked on my whole body, not just my belly, and opened up a new way for me to think about trauma and memory.

Your experiences and memories are remembered by your body. The body has a way of holding and storing the experience in your muscles and organs. Trauma is experienced both physically and emotionally, and, by the time we've lived many years, we have a lot of "memories" held in the body. My stress seemed to always manifest itself in my belly. Most of us know where our stress goes in the body. You might get a stiff neck, have back pain or a spasm, or get headaches.

I learned that I had been holding onto energies that had been created while I was scared and anxious or had suffered trauma, like an accident. The energies remain and need to be released physically and emotionally for the body to function properly and without pain. Sometimes the root cause is so long ago that we don't ever remember it. The original event could have been when you were a baby, and it lives in your body and the subconscious.

After working with her for three sessions, I developed a practice that really helped me. She did not suggest this; it came to me after I learned through her that my past experiences had made me feel unsafe. While I lay in bed every morning, before I even opened my eyes, I would count backwards from 100 while breathing deeply and fully. Filling my belly up with air and totally releasing the breath until nothing was left — that was a count. I would relax and repeat over and over again, "I am safe, I am loved, and I am free."

I knew that the "safe" part was very important, because I never felt safe growing up. It wouldn't have occurred to me that at fifty years old, I still didn't feel safe, or that I had held onto those feelings from when I was young. It started to dawn on me that maybe all the "control" that I tried to enforce throughout my life and on almost everyone in it was to alleviate some of the unsafe feelings. That made so much sense to me, and I really liked repeating "I am safe" over and over. I could feel myself relax as I did it. My body really wanted to hear it. I knew there wasn't a reason to still feel so ill-at-ease. I was as safe as I would ever get. I had to remind myself on a daily basis that I was safe, and it was irrational to feel scared.

The "loved" part was in response to me feeling unlovable for much of my life. I chose to feel unlovable and then I decided to choose differently. My feelings on being and feeling loved have radically changed, and now I firmly believe that we are all loved beyond measure. It was there all the time, but I had to learn it for myself. The love that exists in the Universal Mind or God is a love for each of us as creative, individual parts of the whole and is there for everybody. There is no greater love, and it's never not there. You are loved even if you don't know it or feel it. Next time you feel alone and unloved, check what you're saying in your head. It's a story about why you don't feel loved, but it isn't anything more than what you're choosing to tell yourself.

The "free" part of the prayer was interesting. I didn't understand it at the time. It just came to me, and I went with it. I finally understood that "I am free" is to remind me that we are born with the gift of freedom to choose what we think, how we love, and how we respond. We are free to choose our point of view. Will it be about love and forgiveness or about fear and judgment? Being free to choose is the one thing you can never be stripped of. No matter what happens to you, where you go, or what you do, you can always choose how you think.

Freedom's just another word for happiness.

While growing up in an alcoholic home, I internalized my fear, and as most good type "A" children would do, I put my energies into perfecting the world around me. No matter how good I got at perfecting and doing, I still had the nagging discomfort in my body reminding me that something was wrong. I got used to it — from when I was a little kid until the year of my cancer — I had that pain in my lower left side on a daily basis.

I had the colon resection four weeks after my 34th radiation treatment. The operation went well, and, at the six-week mark, I told my doctor I was still having pain in the same area. He said there is no reason for the pain there. I heard him say, "It's all in your head," even though those were not his words. So, with the last bit of determination I could muster, I started focusing on my left side and giving it the attention it had been demanding for forty years.

There had to be some way of getting rid of the pain by directing my thoughts. I used that prayer/meditation every day for months. I repeated that I was safe, loved, and free.

What I also determined by focusing on the pain was that when I would get into a situation that made me anxious or uptight, I'd hold breath and breathe shallowly. When I started breathing normally, the pain would go away. My breathing was directly connected to the colon pain. After a while, if I consistently took steady, deep breaths, the pain would go away. I don't think I would have been able to "fix" myself without the colon resection, but the pain eventually went away. After forty years of that pain, let me tell you, I was beyond happy.

– 29 –
The Body's Reflexes

I spent quite a bit of time trying to figure out what I was doing with my body unconsciously. While driving the car, I would hold my breath and curl up my toes. How long had I been doing this? I had never thought to pay attention to what I was doing with my body while I drove. My family had joked for years at how awful I was in the passenger seat. It was funny, but also completely true, that I would brace myself on the dashboard of the car the minute someone put the brakes on. I began to check myself in the car to see if I was holding on tightly or relaxed. It became a habit to see how I was breathing, too.

I was in a car accident when I was fourteen, and it was very traumatic. An emergency truck on its way to a fire, going full speed through an intersection, hit our station wagon from the driver's side. Sitting in the front seat next to driver and wearing no seat belt was a combination that made being in a car forever frightening after that. It took six months to recover from breaking every rib, losing my spleen, chipping my teeth, and fracturing my skull. I think that holding my breath and tightening my toes in the car was a learned behavior that didn't get resolved since 1974!

I never paid any attention to what my body was doing or how tight I was holding myself. What I learned from Kerstin was that my body remembered that trauma, and the memories were still there. I began relaxing while I was driving and checking to see how tense I was several times a day. I paid a lot more attention to my breathing and watched how I held myself. I found myself doing things off and on all day, like lifting my shoulders high, pursing my mouth, clenching my jaw, grabbing my thumbs in a fist, breathing half breaths, and tightening my forehead. I wondered if anyone else did things like these.

What was I carrying with me from year to year, maybe since I was young, that affected my health? And I remembered that while growing up, I would always feel sick before school. My mother could never find anything wrong with me. So, after years of dealing with my complaints every morning, she became immune to them, and by first grade, I stopped telling her how nauseous I felt. I learned to live with an anxious feeling before anything I had to do: school, work, appointments of any kind, and especially a trip — this carried into my adult life. But I was so used to it I never even really thought about it — it was just part of "me."

I began to consciously relax all the time, forcing myself to take deep breaths and lower my shoulders. I had never realized how I was holding myself. Now that I knew I was always uptight, it was so much easier to let go. I knew that bracing myself for the next "event," whatever that may be, was from my past experience, and I had to stop — to let my body relax and rest. I did not need to be in protection mode and now I knew that by relaxing I was giving my body the ability to heal itself.

Basically, I had carried all these anxious thoughts and responses with me wherever I went. I had held onto stress from the time I was about seven years old through my adulthood. I buried my anxiety and fear, and all the unresolved emotions, over time, hurt me physically. My unconscious nervousness about what might happen had changed how my body functioned, and all I could do now was realize it and try to keep from doing it in the future.

> "For every effect in our lives, there is a thought pattern that precedes and maintains it. The way we think creates our experiences and by making changes to our thinking patterns, we can change our experiences."
>
> — Louise Hay

Louise Hay wrote a book called *Heal Your Body*. These are the issues that affected me at the time and what she says is the reason:

Abdominal Cramps – Fear. Stopping the process.

Anxiety – Not trusting the flow and the process of life.

Constipation – Incomplete releasing. Holding on to garbage of the past. Guilt over the past.

Nausea – Fear. Rejecting an idea or experience.

And eventually,

Cancer – Deep hurt. Longstanding resentment, deep secret or grief eating away at the self. Carrying hatreds.

After focusing on this for several months, I finally changed the pain in my belly completely, and it hasn't come back. The pain used to be something I would try to ignore (or complain about), but I changed that by focusing on it intensely. That's what my body had been asking me to do. Pain is your body saying, "Notice me!" Now, if I had a pain in my left side, it was because I was reacting to some stress and holding my breath. I would rub my belly, breathe, relax, and feel compassion for my reaction. It changed everything. My pain would be gone within minutes and still is. This was revolutionary for me. What else could I change by refocusing my attention?

– 30 –
Believe It and Become It

I was seven years old when my father got cancer. My parents had four daughters in five years, and their marriage ended when I was nine. It was a violent and overwhelming split for me. When I was twelve, he moved back home to die. He died in the hospital on February 2, 1972. (Coincidentally, February 2 was the day I found out I had breast cancer thirty-eight years later, and the same day I was served with foreclosure papers two years after that.)When he died, he was thirty-seven years old, with four daughters under age twelve. I was totally taken by surprise.

My mother turned to alcohol more and more as I grew up. She was home, but she was in her own world after five o'clock. Her grief was tied up in so many things that it was difficult to figure out what she cried about. She was famous for her crying. After my father died, my mother cried every night for the next ten years.

I had a difficult relationship with her. I tried to control her drinking, coerce her, plead with her, had interventions and arguments, but I was never successful. It was painful for me that she drank, and I never let her forget it.

During my twelfth year, I was molested by our cleaning service. We had four men coming to the house to clean once a week. One day, I was by myself, and they took advantage of that. I was not raped, but I was bruised and frightened. It was shocking that this could happen in my own home, but what happened with my mother would change me forever.

She was angry at me. "What did you do!" I was so taken aback that she wouldn't defend me — it was worse than the event itself. Even worse than her accusation was they were not fired. I had to face them or leave home when they came every week after that. Every time they came back, it reminded me that I wasn't safe in my own house.

When my mother didn't back me up, I lost my safety net. I lost trust in my Universe. This event changed me in ways that I wouldn't be able to see until well into my forties. Basically, my sense of security was so rocked that I felt totally unprotected wherever I went. I worried all the time that if anything happened, I'd have no one to protect me. A lot of my tough, cynical behavior came out of that.

Two years later, I was in the car accident where I was hit by the emergency truck. It was a turning point in my life. The trauma of that accident and the long-term, six month recovery rocked me. I felt completely vulnerable to whatever danger was out there. I never felt safe anywhere after that. I realized how helpless I must have felt at that young age when I became a mother and had kids of my own. If I was untrusting, there were reasons for it. I didn't trust that everything would be okay, because it wasn't. I didn't trust people, because they had let me down and hurt me physically. I had no safe haven, no place of refuge. I was scared in my own house. Scared of what my mother might do, and, even worse, what she wouldn't do to protect me. I was scared of traveling out into the world, in cars, and basically in every aspect of my life. You never would have known it to look at me though. It was all on the inside and I developed a hard shell to keep all my insecurities hidden.

I believed that all this happened because I was unlovable. I was so unlovable that I had to work really hard just to be accepted, let alone loved. If I did everything perfectly, people would really need me and would see that I was worthy of love. I had to work to keep everything under control, so I would be safe. I had to be vigilant — keeping my eye on everything and everybody. I stayed this way for thirty-eight years. I get it now. I get the reasons why I was the way I was. I feel compassion for everyone in the story. I finally can let the story go because I realize that we're all doing the best we can with what we've got. I believe that.

Forgiving my mother has come in waves. Partly because I want no more drama, I try to not mention her in a negative way anymore. Partly because I am a mother and can see where my children blame me for things that I did with love in my heart. And partly because I honor my journey and I wouldn't have had half the learning I've had without my mother's involvement. I was her oldest daughter. I have never laughed harder than I have with my mother. We had a tremendous bond, and when she died, I was relieved that I wouldn't have to be hurt by her anymore but I understand now that that doesn't mean I didn't love her with all my heart.

I ended up marrying someone that I thought would keep me safe. This seems so logical now. I thought he loved me enough that he would protect me and not deceive me. He would shelter me and defend me. I know for a fact I never acknowledged this in my own head, but it was there, under the cover of our marriage. It was a subconscious belief, but it was at the forefront of my reasons for marrying my husband.

We had a good time for many years. We rescued a crazy dog the first year, then we had two kids in fourteen months, and we moved to New Jersey to be near his job. I was working from home and trying very hard to be the mother I didn't have. I thought I was doing a good job. I had been in therapy since I was eighteen, and I continued so I could have help with my kids and my mothering.

I think we were both happy with the way things were, but there was very little depth. Honestly, I don't think I wanted it. Our marriage was not built on knowing each other intimately — we never got to know each other below the surface of daily life. We didn't talk deeply or express ourselves honestly about things that really mattered. It was all fine on the day to day, but when trouble came, we weren't ready for it.

I knew he had lied to me, but I smoothed it over. I would get so mad that I'd threaten to end the marriage, and that just made him better at withholding the truth. I wouldn't let him tell me the truth, because it didn't fit with what I wanted our lives to look like. So I overlooked it.

I began my part in creating a dishonest marriage when I demanded that he act a certain way and to never lie to me. I didn't want a relationship with secrets. That was exactly what I was trying to get away from. There is no safety in secrets, and I wanted to be safe. I wanted him to tell me the truth, and I wanted him to stop doing what he wanted to do. That's how I created dishonesty in my marriage. I'm not saying he didn't do anything to hurt the relationship, but it's obvious what I did to create that.

So instead of looking at the problems head on, I denied them. I made demands, and then denied what was happening beyond that. I was controlling, and I thought that was enough to keep everything in order. The stronger I acted, the more I thought it was going to be fine. Denial was my way to keep feeling safe.

We moved to Rhode Island in 2003 after my husband got fired. There was no reason to stay in New Jersey without his job, and I wanted to be back on the coast. He was badly hurt by losing his job, and he didn't want to go back into the business he had been in so we started a business together. We found a house where we could have retail on the first floor and live on the second and third floors.

Our marriage completely changed when he lost his job. We were falling apart, and I couldn't fix it, so I kept really busy doing things — like working, raising kids and making everything pretty. But even when I didn't have that to do, I'd keep busy doing anything at all to not have to look at us. I was a project queen, with many hobbies and projects to keep busy and feel productive. It was very important for me to feel productive all the time, because that's where I derived my sense of worth. That's how everything stayed together — I was so busy making everything look great that we never had time to look at the truth.

My children were twelve and thirteen when we moved from New Jersey to Rhode Island in the middle of their school year. The stress from the job loss, the switch in states and schools, and starting a new business was high. We actually added to that stress by committing to a house that needed a lot of work.

So here we were in Rhode Island making a new life for ourselves. It sounded like a pretty good scenario to me. Kind of like the great American dream come true, but what was really happening was nothing like that — it was nothing like it could have been. It seemed like such solid plan, but we kept missing the mark. We worked too hard, drank too much, and avoided each other.

We opened the store on my daughter's twelfth birthday. We were in survival mode. Without my husband's corporate job and going into business ourselves, there was a big shift in income. I was exhausted almost all the time. I taught twenty different classes the first month, and we worked 150 days in a row before we closed the store for one day. It was exciting at times and had some high moments, but everything that I had before he got fired was gone. My life that I had built since we got married vanished in one day and was not coming back — I mourned.

After losing his job, he had a lot to prove. He would never take a day off. At one point, we had three girls working the store, and he still wouldn't take a moment off to go do something else. Everything he'd believed about himself had been shaken when he was fired. He wasn't a corporate guy anymore, and if the store didn't do well, he felt it was a reflection of his inadequacies.

The perfectionist in me was extremely busy at this time — it was all I knew how to do to prove I was okay. I was really identified with my abilities, my house, the way I looked, my garden — you name it. My inner voice had an opinion about absolutely everything, and it had an iron grip on me. I was so busy doing what I had to do to keep up that I didn't notice much else. I never took a deep breath. With all my busyness and my dedication to getting things done, I lost my connectedness to myself and my close relationships.

Busyness is a self-imposed distraction.

It's the workings of the ego where, in order to prove your worth, you need to "do." If connection is what turns out to be the most important thing in your life, then spending time being busy and being preoccupied with things to do is a way to waste time. Looking back, it amazes me — the cost to me, my kids, family, friends, and students. We never rested, never took a look at how blessed we were, how much we had to be grateful for and we paid for it in so many ways.

Time went on. We were working hard. The kids were in high school and very involved. The store had been in business for seven years, and I felt like, although we were unhappily married, the business seemed to be okay. We were still working together, but a few years earlier, I had opened a studio in the next town where I went to work and taught jewelry classes. It was not a popular decision to work at another location. He wanted me to be there at the store, but he didn't want to be with me. I think he just wanted to make sure I was working as hard as he was.

I was going to work with a chip on my shoulder every day. Resenting that we didn't talk or have a real partnership, I continued on with a low level of anger underscoring everything. Every six or eight months, I'd complain and demand that we connect somehow. Demanding never worked, but that was all I knew how to do. We agreed on very little. I was surprised to realize that a business created by me, with my ideas and input and working full time at it, could cause me so much unhappiness. But it did. I marched on day after day, feeling resentful and unhappy.

I was pissed about little things all the time, like the laundry that continued to pile up, the lawn not getting mowed, and the garbage not going out. There were a lot of things I felt I had to do that didn't matter. For me, it was easy to confuse a busy life with a rich one.

Just when I thought I couldn't take it anymore — not one more day — I got cancer. There was no coincidence in the "when" of what happened. My underlying desire to get sick was a way to get out of what was going on. I caved and gave up on my life. I got sick and tired. That's what we say — "I am sick and tired of this!" Well, there it is. So I was diagnosed with breast cancer, and I spent a year doing all the things in this book to get back to the life I had given up on.

By the time the year of cancer was over, I had changed so much that there was no turning back. We weren't on different pages; we were in different book stores. He knew it and I knew it. We decided to try marriage counseling, and a part of me held out hope. There's always hope. The way I had been living wasn't working, and I wanted out, but I couldn't throw away twenty-five years. After a year of trying, we sadly let go.

I didn't know that I wasn't privy to the truth of our situation. I just assumed we were where he said we were. We put the house on the market and talked about divorce and selling our business. While we were waiting for the house to sell, the letters came about the foreclosure.

The dynamic way this all unfolded is a testament to the power of what you can create. With what I had in the mix, there was no way to avoid the inevitable fallout. You can't stop that kind of energy — it's too big. You have no choice but to let it play out. At one point, years ago, President Obama used a huge ocean tanker as a metaphor for change. You can't turn a tanker around like a little speedboat. It takes time and distance to make the change in direction.

The degree to which I was able to get through all of what happened is nothing short of a miracle in my eyes — proof that personalities change with every story of growth. My way of dealing with life up until the cancer was through thoughts of control and perfectionism, and the way I dealt with it after that was to keep reminding myself that I didn't know anything for sure. Life was a mystery, and I was just riding the wave and doing the best I could do.

I had spent my life trying to create a safe space. I married for safety and controlled my surroundings for it too. When you spend years trying to avoid deceit, that's exactly what you're going to get. As I said before, the Universe does not distinguish between what you want and what you don't want. It only knows what you're concentrating on. My life came crashing down around me and with the strength I'd found during cancer, I was able to survive it and thrive because of it.

– 31 –
It's Never Finished

C ancer can bring on change faster than you'd ever imagine. If you let it, it can push you like nothing else — igniting a burning desire to get to the core of what matters. Cancer helped me look at my life as an expression of who I truly am and that I can make it what I want. If life begins at the end of your comfort zone — then getting cancer is a way to redefine what it means to live comfortably. I haven't taken a day for granted since I was diagnosed. Comfort is totally overrated — it means little once you've learned how much you want to be here. It gave me a glimpse at my mortality that I would have never opened to.

Life is a continual, shifting, morphing exercise.

Learning that you might not live through the next year brings excitement to that concept. You have a choice every day to celebrate who you are and what you're made of. You are continuously evolving — every minute. Nothing is ever finished regarding your personality or your path. I continue to change and morph into someone new by choice. But we all do; it's just more noticeable with certain people. I don't have the same view I used to have, and, because of that, I act differently — like a completely different person sometimes. It's your choice to be who you are at any given moment.

My life was falling apart, and I understood it was my choice to change or not. My friend Julie turned me on to a new way of looking at my life. My mantra became "I'm not going to do what I've done before." I could choose how I reacted. I could choose when to let go. I could decide to change my story, to forgive at a moment's notice. I could decide to have a different personality. I could dance instead of clean. A type "A" wasn't who I wanted to be anymore — and as Dr. Phil says, "How's that working for ya?" It certainly wasn't working for me either. We have a responsibility to know that our life is up to us. Once we know it and accept it, we can create what we want. The amount of creative expression in your life is up to you.

If and when frustration set in, I just read more, prayed more, and practiced gratitude more. If there is ever a time to test your character, it is when you're really sick. Remember that character is a choice. The longer you act a certain way, the more ingrained it becomes. And this works both ways — for the positive and the negative. Practice enough good feelings and pretty soon you are a positive person. I practice positivity. This is the miracle of learning to train your mind. And it is a miracle. What you thought was your personality — I'm tough, I'm cynical, I'm sarcastic turns into I'm forgiving, I'm understanding, and I'm loving. This is the truth. You become what you think, what you believe, and what you understand to be true.

Once I got cancer, I was able to see how off base I had been. It gave me time to slow down and see where gratitude should have been all along. And so I started to do that: be grateful for a pile of my son's unfolded clothes; be grateful for the opportunity to cry, to laugh, and to see everything from my new perspective. I can choose to see my life from a positive place, no matter what is happening. God, why don't we just do that all the time? All of us...seriously. We have a choice — so choosing a sad story seems like a waste of time, no?

My life as a tough woman was coming to an end. I cried all the time out of gratitude — I still do. I wept at the thought of having the opportunity for another day, and I still do that, too. I try to stay vulnerable with everything. I try to stay gentle. Being grateful is the secret to happiness. Happiness isn't something that happens to you; it's what you find within yourself. Happiness isn't an event; it's what you bring to the event. Any event can be filled with gratitude, because it's only how you view it that makes it what it is. Happiness is completely and 100 percent personal.

I had a newfound patience after the year of cancer. I was not going to give up working on the hard stuff. Losing my guilt, my hardened heart, my lack of trust and critical nature were constant reminders of how far I had come. There was an element, now that I was healthy again, of rebirth. I was free to live a life without these personality traits. In the beginning, I wanted to address them and change just so I wouldn't get cancer again. Now, I wanted to live fully with an open heart and love as my goal day in day out.

As I got gentler and more allowing, my relationships began to change. Questioning myself became the new way to get through the day. "Why did I say that?" "Could I have done that differently?" "Did I show her love?" All day long, trying to change my ancient, locked in behavior was my goal. How much could I open my heart? I would sometimes catch myself and wish I could have done a conversation differently. You don't get a chance to change what you say too often, but if you have an opportunity, you can actually say, "You know, wow, I didn't mean that. What I meant to say was…"

I would look at someone I was talking to, and for the first time in my life, I actually saw them. I understood eye contact as though it was truly "contact." Where had I been looking before? I was seeing people, really seeing them, for the first time in my whole life. Was I so involved with myself I never gave anyone my full attention? I guess I was just so wrapped up in what I was doing that it didn't seem possible to slow down and really listen — I was always thinking, *I'm really busy!* Looking back, I am amazed at the disconnectedness to my life. I just didn't get it. I started listening and connecting with people, paying attention and thinking how amazing it was to finally figure this out.

– 32 –
Being Heard

E xpressing is what we do. There's not a lot of point in expressing ourselves if nobody pays attention. We all want to be heard. To be really understood is probably the most satisfying part of connection. We feel validated and significant. We've all got our own take on what this life means, our reasons and explanations of daily interactions, relationships, histories, and to have someone really hear what you have to say is a gift. When you speak your piece, especially when it's something you feel is important, the best thing anyone can do for you is to listen.

When it's your turn to listen, try seeing beyond what is being said and relate to someone on a more intuitive level. Not just because it's kind and giving, but because hearing someone is more than just words. The most profound thing you can do for someone is to listen without an agenda. To listen to someone without thinking of what you want to say next (so you can sound smart) is the nicest, most loving way to make someone feel understood. Open your heart along with your ears. Try to hear what they're really saying. Listen and feel what they have to say — hear beyond the words into the meaning and intent.

Don't think about what you want to say in response. Don't think of ways to help. Don't think about what you can do for them or chime in with your ideas. Don't think about anything else — just listen to what they're telling you. Feel and hear what they want you to understand. It's something we don't usually do. You'll see, when you think you are paying attention, you don't normally put all of your attention onto the conversation. You are thinking of two or three other things at the same time. But if it's our greatest gift, couldn't we make a better effort? If we all just want to be heard and to be truly seen, isn't that a wonderful way to show someone how much you love and honor who they are?

Look with more than your eyes; include your heart when you look, feeling with your heart, sensing the struggle in all of us to be loved and heard. We are all one. No one is above this. All of us, no matter who we are, are above wanting to be loved and understood. We are here to communicate and express our uniqueness. Connection is what we're after — whether you believe it or not — that's where you get what you're looking for. So connecting with everyone you know — whether it's on a very small level with the person you're standing in line with or your partner of twenty-five years — is where life's meaning comes from. The best part of everyday can be the times when you gave yourself completely to an interaction and you didn't even have to say a word.

Learning the importance of my interactions with people has been the biggest blessing of my life. I used to think it was all about me. I used to think that I was the center of my Universe. The part that shifted for me was when I understood that even though I'm at the center of my Universe, my contribution relates to everyone else. If I am really listening to you and giving you my undivided attention, then I'm creating a sense of well-being in you — a sense of importance and relevance. That's what I have to give that matters.

There was a part of me that wanted to avoid true connection, because I was scared of being judged unworthy and unlovable, as well as the potential pain of not measuring up. I still struggle with this, but, as each interaction comes and goes, I learn that being vulnerable and honestly connected can only help me grow to empower myself and other people. My intent is to really understand and open to what you have to share with me. If it's easy to hear you, I still listen with the same attention as if it were very involved and complicated. I try to listen with the same intensity, no matter what you want to share. Interacting with people is what my life is about now.

– 33 –
Losing Self-Consciousness

When I was able to go back to work, I felt energized. My classes were completely different than the ones I'd taught before. I didn't think about how I sounded or what the students thought of me. That's the difference between being self-conscious and finding consciousness. I only thought about what I could do for them. As a teacher, I always thought about my responsibility to impart information and help people understand what I was trying to teach. A completely different approach formed when I came back to work after cancer.

I didn't care so much about the information anymore. I knew I had a point to make and had to help people understand what they needed to learn, but it became secondary. Now, my main concern was seeing the students. I mean seeing them as they are — as individuals. Not that I didn't care about what they were learning, of course I did, but it wasn't my main concern anymore. I wanted to connect, because I loved connecting. I think when I taught classes before, I was so wrapped up in myself that it distracted me. My image, my delivery of the lesson, my feelings about the class, whatever I was thinking, it was mostly about me — my ego was totally attached to me as the teacher. What would the class think of my lesson? Would they think I was a good teacher? Did I look good today? Everything I thought of was based on me and my insecurities and fears. My new focus had nothing to do with how I appeared to the class — it's so amazing now to see it — my focus was on the students themselves.

If you truly believe in loving everyone and concentrating on the good in everyone, giving everyone an "A", you can seriously clear your body of any preoccupation and feel free and complete just the way you are. Your concern for your appearance and how you measure up falls away. When this feeling began to take over, my classes changed tremendously.

If I take the energy to really engage in what you're about and what you're trying to tell me, then I don't have the ability to concentrate on myself and what I'm about. If I spend my time paying attention to you and hear what you have to say, my energy is so focused on you that I lose my self-centeredness – it doesn't mean I don't engage, it just means I'm more connected to the conversation. Without my self-centeredness, I'm not conflicted with other thoughts that take away from me hearing you and being present. I can be in the present moment concentrating on you. What a difference this makes! Is there any better way to spend my time? Giving myself to the people around me by just staying focused and letting go of my ego is how to live fully in the moment.

174

– 34 –
What's Focus Got to Do with It?

U sing your power to create the life you want is all about your focus. Learning to train your attention to what you want is easy, but you have to be relentless. Keeping track of thousands of thoughts an hour might be impossible, but catching the damaging, negative ones that repeat over and over merely takes commitment. You can use your energy wisely, or you can expend it on thoughts that do you no good. You are actively bringing into existence what you think about all day long.

Being focused on what you don't want is just like asking it to come your way. The energy you create with thoughts has nothing to do with a yes or no energy. It's the same energy. So, in other words, if you focus on having no money and not wanting to be poor, you're still focused on poverty. The energy doesn't distinguish between wanting and not wanting. It just focuses on what you're thinking about. The energy is being emitted and creating the situation. So even though you don't want it, you're bringing it all right to you. You cannot focus on unwanted things to get to what you want.

When I got married, I partly chose a man that I trusted completely specifically because I didn't want deceit, and it was absolutely that same energy that brought me to my knees in lies. If I believed I was unlovable, and I married fearing this, that's what I was and what I became. I feared for my financial security, which manifested in financial ruin. I didn't want chaos, and that's what I ended up with.

You have incredible power, and realizing this is the key.

Your power is all in your mind, but it has to be trained. Watching your thoughts takes awareness and perseverance. Your power is not hard to feel, to realize. It seems like a stretch to say, "I have power." You might think, *Where is it? I can't feel it or find it.* But it's always there. All the time. You never don't have it. You just need to focus it to see it working.

Tapping into your power only takes a moment — holding onto it requires skill and focus. It's easy to be distracted by the life going on around you. Feeling your power is feeling the moment you're in. Your power isn't found tomorrow or in forty-five minutes, or when you're ready — it's now.

If you sit still and focus on your body and your breathing, you can feel your power. Your body hums, your mind is expectant, and you are right here waiting on the brink in this moment. That is power. If you are here, right now, without your story, your power is available. Being un-conflicted and focused is how you concentrate on your power.

Part of your power comes from taking responsibility for your life on a moment-by-moment basis, staying with yourself when it would be easy to numb out or what I call split off. When you split off from yourself, you reject your power. Part of what you feel when you want to numb out is your energy and power that needs to be released. Sometimes you feel uneasy sitting in the moment — that's your energy making you uneasy. That uneasiness or restlessness is the energy inside of you. See it for what it is and embrace it.

> "Our deepest fear is not that we are inadequate. Our deepest fear is that we are powerful beyond measure. It is our light, not our darkness that most frightens us. We ask ourselves, 'Who am I to be brilliant, gorgeous, talented, fabulous?' Actually, who are you not to be?"
> — Marianne Williamson,
> *A Return to Love: Reflections on the Principles of "A Course in Miracles"*

It doesn't have to be a feeling you want to escape from. When you name it as power or your energy, it is easier to hold it. Sit with it and feel it. If you can rest here with it, your energy can be healing and open to anything you want. When you attach thoughts to this feeling of energy, you can misunderstand it. The only way to understand it is to be with it; you can't put words to it easily. You can't look for it, because it's always there. It's impossible to find, because it's never not available.

You might feel compelled to distract yourself from this feeling of power. Addictions come from this wanting to escape yourself. You could say you feel bored and reach for something to undo the boredom, but it's not boredom, it's just mislabeling the moment right now. Trying to escape from it doesn't do a thing to alleviate the boredom or uneasiness — it just saves it for another time.

When I feel my energy level in excess, and I call it this instead of anxiousness, restlessness, or boredom, I find a way to release. I can put my focus on ways to release some of my power. The loving and nurturing way to get through an anxious state is to name it and embrace it — not run away from it. If you understand that this is your power, you are less likely to try and struggle away from it. Instead, I choose to work with it and release it when I feel too much. If I can sit in it and wait with it, concentrating on my positive thoughts and putting my energy where it'll help me, that's the best way of using power.

Built up energy and anxiety can lead you to want to act out in ways that are destructive. Feeling your power in those moments is difficult, because you aren't used to facing it. Checking out — eating when you're not hungry, watching TV, shopping, drinking, gambling, these are all ways to prolong and avoid facing that energy. You might try to avoid your power, because it feels like too much to hold. Feeling it can be overwhelming. Focus on what it is — don't try to get away. It's just you at full strength. Your power is your body and mind coming together in the moment without a story going on.

"The most common way people give up their power is by thinking they don't have any."

— Alice Walker

The power that's yours is present whenever you are focusing on the moment. In that moment, you are not thinking about other moments — past or future. You have everything you need in this moment. You are breathing, you are feeling what is happening in your body, in your head — you are aware. Feel the power. It isn't complicated; rather, it's full of potential.

The present moment is full of infinite potential.

When you're making decisions, having conversations, listening to people, and doing what you do, you are focused and not conflicted — all of these things are completely different experiences when you're in your place of power. Letting go of your ego is where this begins. There's no story when you're in the moment, so you're free to access your true energy.

Experiencing really difficult times, like getting diagnosed with cancer, can be a "powerful" experience. If you can hold the moment, make space for the moment, and let it sit there, you can act powerfully. The way you handle new information is important. Breathing, concentrating on being present, listening, and feeling acceptance of what's happening holds the space for peace and power.

– 35 –
Preparing for Power

B racing yourself for appointments or situations that could be stressful is very helpful. Bringing quietness into your body, preparedness, and calmness when you have medical procedures helps your body-mind tremendously. Staying right in the moment, without projecting what might happen or thinking about what has happened in the past, keeps your power focused and lets your body do what it needs to do without distraction. Worrying about what might happen or dwelling on past experiences takes your power away and keeps you in the protection mode.

Think of your power as having all of you as a whole, available right now in the present. This means no distractions or projections, nothing taking your attention away — it's you at your highest, best, and most focused. Your energy can be trained, so it's concentrated on one thing. If you're in a doctor's office and having a conversation, and you aren't preparing what to say while they're talking, you aren't analyzing while they're explaining, you aren't giving advice or interjecting, then you're listening from a place of power. This is putting your power to use and can affect what you take away from the conversation.

When I'm truly focused, I've experienced moments of concentrated power where I'm completely undivided and totally present. The only way to do this is to dismiss the dialogue in your head. You have nothing to defend or uphold. You are free to believe that you and this moment are absolutely perfect in every way, and there's no need to alter anything. There's nothing to have a story about. There's no need for an angle or opinion. Make a conscious decision not to defend or justify before you begin a conversation, and this frees the moment up for expansion.

The way to take charge of your life is to first and foremost understand that you are responsible for all of it. You have created everything you see in your world. What you focus on is what you become, and this is true for all the events in your life. Nobody makes your life but you. No one takes care of you but you. I don't mean this in just the physical sense, because I'm also talking about your way of thinking. How you think and use your power is how you create your life. When you focus, you can calm, prepare, manage, and align your body.

You're responsible for your happiness on all levels. Nobody can live your journey or take a part of your journey. It's your journey, and, like it or not, even if somebody else is supporting you or taking care of you, it's still up to you to be responsible for your own happiness. You either accept that you're in control or not. Holding the vision of what you want your life to look like, staying in control of your view point, and keeping a steady focus on what's important will bring you happiness and well-being.

When something in your life goes wrong, and you're faced with a painful situation, one of the hardest but most effective things to do is to see where you were in it. What part did you play — honestly? Where was your heart leading up to what happened? Were you trying to manipulate, ignore, or control? Get real about your part. This is power at its greatest — to be honest about your contribution. Don't be afraid to see what you did or said to add to what happened. How else can you learn and grow? Feeling that things are happening to you makes it all out of your control. You have control when you are present and honest. If that's what you want, stay there. Drop out of your story and look at your truth. It's hard looking at truth but that's where you get to grow.

The question you have to ask yourself is: do you want to be someone out of control or do you want to be in the flow? I'm not saying that things won't happen outside of your plan — I'm saying when they do, you are going to be in a completely different place mentally, emotionally, and spiritually. Nothing is part of a story anymore; it's just the truth. That in itself gives you power. When you hold yourself steady, grounding your energy, you'll feel the control of your life come back.

If someone is accusing you of certain behavior and you flatly deny it, take another look. Denying what is seen in you is usually a way to defend or pretend. Try to look at the situation from the other perspective and see what it is they're seeing. Is there truth there? Even a little bit of truth will inspire growth. Is it painful to see what they see? If it's painful, it's worth looking at. There's usually truth in what people notice about you. How can you learn from it? Denying and defending does you no good. Defending behavior isn't the way to learn — it's a waste of time. If you did what you thought was appropriate, you wouldn't need to defend it. If you feel you have to argue, it's a great time to really see where you stand and what you're trying to accomplish.

There is a big difference between becoming aware of your energy and actualizing it. Believing in it and living it are two different things. Putting into practice what you believe in takes dedication and determination. Awareness of yourself can be painful and difficult, because you might not always like what you see. There's a pretty good chance you're not looking for awareness if you're blissfully happy without it; searching for the truth about yourself usually comes because you're in pain. But seeking and discovering the truth about you can be more life-changing than anything else. The more behavior you're willing to notice and learn from, the more you can hold your sense of peace.

Who am I to choose what I should and should not experience? Who's to say I shouldn't have pain in my life? I try to give thanks for my blessings and my struggles with the same amount of energy, because without one I can't appreciate the other. It's all good. Staying vulnerable and open to life can be tenuous at times. Parts of the old me are afraid of being hurt, but the new part of me says, "Bring it on!" Pain? So what? Pain and pleasure are two sides of the same coin. You can't get to the one without risking the other. There's nothing bad about pain. The Inner Eye looks at pain with the same kind of detached witnessing as it does with pleasure. Life is full of both. Don't dismiss your life experience trying to avoid pain, because without that contrast, you lose the pleasure. Knowing that without pain you don't know pleasure is very powerful.

Sometimes a little quiet and concentration is extremely beneficial. Pulling yourself together to center yourself gives you strength and purpose. We all get caught up and distracted with living. Before anything you have to do, whether it's an appointment or a cup of coffee, stop and gather yourself. Breathe a deep breath. Gather your gentleness and trust. Remember what you want and who you want to be — kind, loving, and allowing. This helps to prepare you for anything.

– 36 –
Personality

P ersonality and character are a choice. If you want to have good character, you can make it happen — it is not something solid and permanent that you can't change. Saying that people don't change is just not true. It is ridiculous to say that you are a certain way — "That's just the way he is," or "I was born like that." That's absolute nonsense. Saying that you do something because of your personality is an excuse to defend your behavior. Your personality is just a way you've acted over and over to make a pattern. That pattern becomes what you think you are — who you are. It's not who you are; it's just a pattern of behavior.

If you decide to do something differently, does that mean you're a different person? No, you've made a shift in behavior. People change all the time — we change daily. Your body, your thoughts, what you choose to believe changes. It's inevitable that we change and daily, if not hourly.

If you get a speeding ticket, you change your behavior and slow down. If you get a rash when you eat something, you don't eat it anymore. When you get cold, you put a sweater on. If you decide to act differently because you have a new understanding, you don't say your personality has changed; you say you've changed your mind or learned something new. That's what lessons are all about. What changes is how you respond to a situation. It might be a big, fundamental shift, or just deciding not to get into the same argument again. Your actions are your choice, so your "personality" is too.

We all have a belief of who we are. I believed I was strong and I took the time and effort to prove it all the time. My personality was bold and outspoken. I played into my personality because it played into my story, but that's all it was. Being headstrong has gotten me into some amazing situations. I always thought that I knew what I was doing. I always thought that I could handle what was happening. I believed that I could make life happen, and I didn't want life to take me where I didn't want to go. I thought I could use my personality to control the situation.

What I believed about my personality encouraged me to act in certain ways. If you change the perception of yourself and open to being other than that, you can be anyone you want to be.

Believe in what you want to be, not in what you think you are.

Remind yourself what you'd like to be and act that way. Your personality has nothing to do with how you act or what you can be. It's how you've been programmed up until you decide to be different. Your actions and responses are totally in your control. If you want to be gentle, and you'd like to be more understanding, then think of yourself that way. You'll end up being that way.

I used to repeat a couple of sentences every day, all day long, when I had cancer – hundreds and hundreds of times. "I am kind, gentle, and allowing. My thoughts, words, and actions are healthy and uplifting. I happily contribute wherever I can." This was a new way of thinking for me. I wanted to believe it, and I repeated it whenever I could. These were "personality" traits that I wanted. I believed that I could have them if I wanted them.

I have learned that the opposite of making life happen is allowing life to unfold. This is a hard lesson for someone who did a lot of controlling. I now trust that this is the best way. Talk about twisting my arm — this has not come easily to me. Changing your personality, just like changing your mind, does not come easily. Once I stopped controlling all the time, the allowing started to happen on its own. Allow things to happen. Allow people to make mistakes. Allow relationships to change. Let people see you the way they want to. Let your control go, and your stress goes away. Do not insulate yourself from the pain of uncertainty. Be uncertain — it will make you grow.

I believe that letting go of control and allowing things to unfold could be the best health advice there is. Struggling with life is hard, and it saps your energy and strength — not to mention, you don't have as much power over events as you might think. It's unhealthy to fight with life. It becomes easier to let go the more you do it.

Going with the flow is the way that nature keeps her strength, like how a tree bends in the wind or a river finds the easiest route. Trust is one of my biggest lessons in this life, and the best way to practice your trust is to let go. I don't want to be dragged; I'm going to let go.

I think we come here to learn and grow with love. I believe we are here for a purpose. I also believe that we are part of a fabulous plan. I think the Universe is a loving one, and, through love, we are urged to learn about ourselves and stretch beyond what we thought we could be. Growing can be painful and it isn't easy or relaxing, but what better way to spend your time? We're not here to just sit.

When I get to the end of my life, I will say that I gave it my best. I tried, I grew, I learned, and I loved the best I could. I stayed when I wanted to leave, and I left when I could have stayed all in the name of growth. I will not waste time avoiding my truth just so I can be comfortable — I don't have time to avoid myself. This is my emotional journey so I'm going for all the emotion there is. Let me see what's there and have the grit for it – why not? Because it's uncomfortable? I'd rather use my time here for what's uncomfortable and get to a new understanding of myself than sit back and avoid my lessons. Learning about me is what I'm here to do.

I developed perfectionistic traits at a young age. They were the result of my way of coping. I have spent much of my life being critical, because being perfect is impossible. You absolutely can't do it — therein lies the built-in criticism. I was mostly critical of myself, but you can't be accepting of others if you're critical of yourself.

Just know that it's true — if you are judging yourself, you're judging everyone else, too.

I didn't agree with this for a very long time. I felt compassion and understanding and I thought I was an accepting person. It is impossible to be truly accepting of others if you spend time putting yourself down. On many levels, you will criticize other people if you can't accept your own imperfections. True acceptance starts with you, and you cannot be accepting if you're critical.

The true test of compassion is when you can show it to yourself.

If you can't show yourself compassion, then there is no way that you're compassionate to others. You might act compassionately, but below the surface is a judgment. Acceptance and allowing is what a spiritual journey is all about, and reaching for it is a practice, not something you get to and are done.

I have a great understanding and love for perfectionists. Your ego has convinced you that's how to survive and be loved. It's the idea that you aren't good enough just as you are — you must work at perfecting everything to gain acceptance and belonging. It's so difficult to live in that role — my heart swells when I recognize a fellow perfectionist. There should be a twelve-step program for us. I did it for such a long time that it's a hard act to break. To believe that you have to perform perfectly to be accepted is what sets the perfectionist apart.

"Understanding the difference between healthy striving and perfectionism is critical to laying down the shield and picking up your life. Research shows that perfectionism hampers success. In fact, it's often the path to depression, anxiety, addiction, and life paralysis."

— Brene Brown

When I got around to looking at my critical nature, it was overwhelming. I had spent a lifetime being right, being the best, or at least thinking I was close to it and proving myself day after day —performing at levels that were exhausting. It took a lot of work — always trying to be the person I had decided I needed to be instead of just being the person that was already here. It was sucking the life out of me, but I was so busy powering through, I didn't notice.

Being critical causes a lot of guilt. You can't judge someone without creating guilt. You don't consciously feel the guilt, your ego won't let you, but it's there. Judging is what the ego does to justify itself. I judge you to make me feel better, stronger, and smarter. The ego makes sure that we come out on top by judging and comparing to bolster our opinion of ourselves. Every thought about someone else that is not accepting is a judgment. Even saying something like, "She's having a hard time," is a judgment. It's difficult to have an average conversation without judging, because we don't typically watch what we say and think.

In *The Four Agreements*, Miguel Ruiz lists the four things that if you practice, will bring your ego in check.

The four agreements are: don't take anything personally; don't make assumptions; always do your best; and be impeccable with your word.

Being impeccable with your word is, in my mind, the most difficult. Not so much from the outside, but from the inside. You know when you say something judgmental. You can curb your comments, and although it takes a lot of practice, the rewards are stunning. No guilt, no bad feelings, no regret — just be impeccable with your word.

The difficult part is keeping your thoughts impeccable as well. Finding the balance between observing what you're thinking and actually engaging and believing in your thoughts is crucial to your health. When you choose to criticize yourself or someone else and keep it in your own mind, it still creates guilt. The guilt that you hold will always come back to bite you in one form or another. It leaves a heaviness in your body. And once you're aware of that feeling, it becomes noticeable whenever you create it. Guilt is something that builds from day to day, and we get used to the feelings it produces. We get so used to it that it feels normal.

Learning to love myself changed my personality. In many cases, learning to love yourself will bring back your health. When we can learn to love ourselves to the point that our inner voices are kind, gentle, and caring, there is the possibility for much greater love in our relationships. The constant beating up of ourselves is so counterproductive. We all know this, but do we stop? You have to train your mind to stop it. Where there is love on the inside, there'll be love on the outside.

Where there is criticism on the inside, there'll be judgment on the outside.

I was always criticizing myself for my behavior, for my body, for my thoughts. I worked really hard at stopping. I consciously worked at being kind, because I knew that if I couldn't be kind to me, how could I be kind to others?

At one point, I was beating myself up for gaining five pounds, like it was something that wasn't supposed to happen again. I was so disappointed in myself. Doesn't everyone go through this? But I was hearing the "voice" that makes me feel like a failure and definitely not okay. I'd finally had enough. I cut it right off and said kindly, "It's okay, really. Your weight does not determine your worth. You'll get the weight off when you're ready." This voice had such a sweetness to it that it almost made me cry. I didn't recognize it. I was starting to feel compassion for myself, and it was new for me. I guess I'd had enough of that angry voice. There was no question which one I would rather pay attention to. When you pay attention to the kinder voice, it'll grow and so do you. When you're kinder to yourself, you're kinder to everyone.

Changing the voices in your head is a choice, just like your personality. As with everything else in the mind, you can choose to accept it or choose to reject it. It's the thoughts that we think over and over again that become who we think we are. But that just isn't true; that's only who we THINK we are. You are not your thoughts. You might identify with some of them, but they are not you.

Creating good thoughts is a necessary part of changing the inner critical voice, and, in turn, your character. If I am criticizing myself for gaining weight, how is that really going to help me? Criticism doesn't do much for motivation other than shame you into action.

I don't know about you, but I'd like to avoid shame and guilt if I can.

Making me feel bad doesn't help and will NOT be the reason I get my act together and lose the weight. When you are nurturing with yourself, you'll stay in touch with your inner Self. Criticism tends to make you split off from yourself and disassociate with what's going on.

Instead of shaming me into eating less and exercising more, I can say what I know I would like to hear. "Kim, you are capable of whatever it is that you want to do. Relax!" We all know how to lose weight. When you get caught up in the new diet fad or trying something different, it just takes more concentration and distracts you from what you should be doing — which is living, loving, and growing. I don't want to waste my precious energy on losing weight anymore, and, even more importantly, being critical of myself.

> "For some reason, we are truly convinced that if we criticize ourselves, the criticism will lead to change. If we are harsh, we believe we will end up being kind. If we shame ourselves, we believe we end up loving ourselves. It has never

been true, not for a moment that shame leads to love. Only love leads to love."

— Geneen Roth

A voice that promotes good feelings is a lot healthier to listen to. I don't want to hear any negativity. I am done with that, especially if the thought is from within and nobody else can hear it. My heart is beating for me. It's on my side. My body is a reflection of what I am thinking and feeling. I want those feelings to be good. I want to be impeccable with my word and my thoughts, because it feels good — NOT because I want to be perfect. I want peace and happiness even when I'm talking to myself.

Choose what you want to say to yourself. It is a choice to feel peaceful and uplifted. I don't have to listen to what my ego is trying to tell me. I know it's hard to get around the ego, but once you get an idea of how tricky and persistent it can be, you're on the right track. We all have to learn to disregard the critical inner voice. It's a waste of time, and it's not good for our bodies — it is absolutely not healthy.

Lighten up! Be free of destructive behavior and reach your full potential — stop doing the things that hold you back. Change your thinking.

We are free to choose:
1. Happiness over sadness/anxiety
2. Contentment over loneliness
3. Love over fear
4. Peace over control
5. Interest over boredom
6. Gratitude over expectations

– 37 –
Goodness

"In order that the mind should see light instead of darkness, so the entire soul must be turned away from this changing world, until it's eye can bear to contemplate reality and that supreme splendor which we call the good."

— Socrates

I believe there is a larger purpose evolving in all life. It's life learning about itself. Seemingly random events are connected by layers of purpose. We will never have the distance to see what everything means, so I have faith and the belief in goodness to keep moving forward with a positive viewpoint. This is the primary thought that I live by — the belief in goodness.

Believing in the goodness behind every situation enables you to remain allowing. If you believe in goodness, letting go becomes easy. You let go a little bit all the time, because you believe all is well. When you stop clinging to things, your fear of lack lessens, because you're not holding on. If you have nothing to hold onto, you're free.

When I feel myself clinging to an outcome, I have to ask myself why.

Depending on an outcome to have happiness will never work, because you're dependent on something outside of yourself and therefore out of your control. Your peace and happiness are always in your control, because they're coming from within you. When you let your belief in goodness override your fear of lack, you're free to allow things to unfold.

The difference between clinging and allowing is that by allowing, you let go of your thought of control. You take the "I" out of the equation, which puts you in the passenger seat instead of the driver's seat. Just because you aren't driving doesn't mean you won't get to where you want to go. Being a passenger doesn't mean you don't make decisions; it just means that when you do, you're open to the driver's route as well. Letting go opens you up to more options and eventualities. How do you know that you're not clinging to the wrong thing? If you're attached less to the outcome, you can keep a better perspective on all situations and make better decisions.

Your perception is always incomplete. We seldom stop to think about how little we know. We are so bent on being in charge, knowing the answer and deciding what is right. If we don't know something, we feel less intelligent. Sometimes not knowing is the smarter approach. Judging situations based on what we know is always incomplete. We view a situation or experience, and then decide what we think is right or wrong. This is totally unnecessary. We don't need to make a judgment.

All judgments are incomplete.

You can replace your anxious thoughts with thoughts of goodness. Think about a chance meeting with the perfect person, timing being just right to find what you were looking for, a surprise of great fortune, and amazing coincidences that bring you to the places you want to be. The potential for goodness is unending.

Believe in the miraculous.

Here's a question for you: why not? There are many ways to look at situations, and being anxious is only one way. Think of all the other ways and change your mind — turn it around. Go for the thought that makes you smile instead. If you could go either way, why wouldn't you go for good news? If you're projecting anyway, why not project something positive.

Positive thinking is being able to face reality and choose the viewpoint that looks to goodness. This is not unrealistic thinking. This is choosing to see goodness. You are not at the mercy of your environment — you have a choice every minute of every day — where will you hold yourself? Above and responsible for your part or below, waiting to see what awful things happen next. Believing in goodness has nothing to do with denial — it has to do with taking the high road.

When I was in the middle of my cancer ordeal, I would repeat over and over the same thing — going into surgery, having the chemo put into my port, driving to the hospital — all the time: "I know and trust that only good comes to me." I release all my feelings of control, knowing that only good is happening — no matter what it is. I believe in the goodness of everyone around me and all things.

Goodness is a choice. Your viewpoint can start with goodness and go from there. It's possible to find the good in any situation, but we don't always do that. We forget. This is absolutely a daily practice — finding the good — and it's not hard — it's an exercise.

When you want to get strong, you work out every day and you become stronger over time. It takes time. The same with believing in goodness. Build your strength to find the good. Make finding goodness a daily practice. You can find good in places you never knew, but until you start trying to see it, you won't find it. It's an internal muscle that needs exercise. Sometimes it's not just your viewpoint — it's searching for something that hasn't been seen yet, or just knowing that it's there even if you can't see it. Believe and trust that it's all good.

Why is it so important to find the good in things? The shift to finding goodness in everything instead of seeing the opposite is a life-changer. I believe that my time is spent on a totally different level when I'm above life's negative fray. If I can live in a place of peace and kindness (the good), how much better will my life be? If I have a choice, why would I choose otherwise?

Also, it feels great. Feeling great is good for your health. Finding good and then feeling good is as healthy a way to spend your day as you can get. Feeling good spreads love and gratitude — the healthiest of emotions. If you feel good, it's hard not to spread it around. Spreading a good feeling around is where joy comes in.

Joy is something you're open to. Knowing it's there is half of it. Most people wouldn't say they experience joy on a daily basis, but are they looking for it? If I want joy in my life, I need to create it and be ready for it. It is totally within my ability to bring joy to me. Be open to goodness, and joy comes into your life. Gentleness, kindness, and joy are all forms of goodness.

When I was younger, I had no idea that you could create good feelings yourself. I thought I had to wait until they came to me. I thought that goodness was out there somewhere, but it wasn't within reach. Some people had it and some didn't. Now I know it's in my control to feel it. Maybe some of us were born with good things and some of us weren't, or maybe it's just a way of seeing your life. I didn't think it was something I could make happen.

But what if I were taught that it was the way I looked at my life? What if believing in goodness and seeing it all around us is the way to bring it to you? What if we taught children that they could make their lives filled with goodness by just believing in it? You absolutely can make good things happen by feeling good and seeing good. It's within your ability to create it.

You do not become good by trying to be good, but by finding the goodness that is already within you and allowing that to come through. Discover goodness everywhere you look. Believe in your own goodness. Know that without a doubt you are good. But also, no matter how hard it may seem, believe in all our goodness — even people who don't seem to want to be good.

> "All my life, I have wanted to lead people to an empathy space, to a gratitude space. I want us each to be awake to our full potential, to find our calling, and to summon the courage to live it. Imagine a world where we all lift ourselves up, and then reach out and lift someone else. And so together, we rise."
>
> — Oprah

Where you put your focus is where your life goes. If you put your focus on goodness, love, and positive point of view, it is where your life will go. It has no other option. There is nothing that can happen that you won't see differently when you're focused on goodness. Your focus and attention can create anything you desire, so remember that when you are thinking negative thoughts.

Here's the thing, seriously. If you have a choice and we are all free to choose, then why not choose goodness, love, and positive point of view? What are your other options? Drama, stress, sadness, and ego-driven stories? You can let life happen to you — to react — to be the victim in your life or you can make the choice to see everything differently. This is a choice, you understand. You choose your thoughts — you pick the thoughts that you agree with, and then you operate around them. Accept this as truth, and it is yours.

– 38 –
Viewpoint

I felt I had a pretty good chance of getting cancer in the first place. My father, mother, and grandfather had all died from it. There was always the possibility that I would end up like them, and, because my parents died young, I had a lot of time to think about that fact — years of thinking about it. I always knew it was a possibility, and that was exactly the thinking that helped bring it into existence.

I realized that I had brought cancer to me. I actually took years to bring it to me, and I managed to set the stage for it perfectly. After my father died when I was twelve, I used to calculate that I had a one in four chance of getting cancer. This was my own math, and I was only twelve, but I thought that because I had three sisters, one of us would get cancer, and it could definitely be me. Then, when I was thirty-one, my mother died of cancer, and that solidified the fact that it was a very real possibility. My viewpoint was going to make the outcome pretty easy.

That thinking alone was hardly enough to make it happen, but I worked on other things as well. Along with the belief that I would someday have cancer, I held onto resentments, hardly ever forgave a betrayal, and kept track of rights and wrongs done to me. I thought this was normal, and I was always envious of people who let things slide. How did they forgive so easily? It baffled me. Forgiveness never came naturally to me, and I saw no great reason to work on it. I could defend all my actions with really good reasons to stay hurt. That's how I kept my story going — maintaining all the right arguments for keeping all my hurt and resentments alive. My viewpoint was from a place of lack and fear.

The bottom line is that I have a choice to bring sadness, illness, and misfortune to me with my viewpoint. If I choose to believe in negative things happening, they will. When I hold onto resentments and the wrongs done to me, my viewpoint is totally limited to that energy. Thinking that way limits the happenings in my life to negative experiences. If forgiveness, goodness, and gentleness are the way I live, then I'm open to everything and everyone. No limits then. One way of living is closed, and the other is open. One viewpoint is expansive, and the other is limited.

Being able to change your thoughts is the single most powerful tool that you have.

And I learned about that when I had cancer. It's so simple. You are in charge of your mind and the thoughts you choose to keep there. The ideas that come and go are not yours — and especially, they are not a reflection of you. There is no way to keep them from coming to you. This phenomenon is a universal part of being human, and to try to control it is impossible. You can, however, put as much or as little emphasis on your thoughts as you want. A thought comes into your head, and you say, "Oh, interesting thought," and let it go. Then another comes and it's more insistent. "Look, another thought, big deal," and you treat it like it was nothing. You don't have to force anything, you just don't pay attention to the thoughts that don't fit the "you" that you want to be.

When I looked at my actions — the way I was living my life — I was putting a lot of emphasis on what wasn't right. I was thinking that things should be a certain way, and when they weren't, I wasn't happy. My view of my life, my story that I told myself, was all about what I didn't want. My thoughts about my life were the wrongs. Nothing was wrong in my life, but my thoughts about it made it seem wrong. I chose to hold onto and emphasize thoughts that were about negativity. It was my choice. It was a story I was telling myself. I talked myself into that story every day. I defended it and nurtured it with my beliefs.

If my health depends to a great extent on how I perceive my life, then I will choose to view it with love and gratitude. If my happiness is dependent on what I think about, then I'll be sure to think about what is going well and what I have to be thankful for. If the general reality of my existence is up to me and what thoughts I choose, then I will choose the thoughts that make me happy. This is my choice. When you know that you can choose, your options are limitless.

Your point of view is everything in this life.

It's as simple as having a happy life or not, and it's all about choice. How you view your experience is up to you, and you make up your mind to choose what you want to think. It comes down to awareness — the awareness of yourself and what you're thinking. Your point of view is a decision. If you choose to accept thoughts that are negative, then that's the experience you'll have.

The moral of the viewpoint story is it's never as it seems — EVER. You just don't know anything for sure. You know a tiny little bit of what goes on in your surroundings. Basically, you're in the dark. As long as you know you're in the dark, you can give all your judgments and opinions on the subject away. If you aren't given all the information, which you never are, then you can't come up with a realistic answer to "why," so don't even try. You create your viewpoint from a place of innocence. You create your viewpoint from a place of goodness, kindness and compassion. You make no judgments because they are not yours to make.

If we assume the point of view that we really have no idea about what goes on in other people's lives, we won't judge. We don't know what they're exposed to, what they experience, what they think about. From day to day, we are all exposed to so many things. We become different people all the time. Any kind of judging or assuming we do about someone else is totally ridiculous. How could we know enough to make a fair judgment? It's impossible. And by the way, what is a fair judgment? According to whom? Me? Nobody can be a fair judge on any subject. A judgmental viewpoint is limiting, and that creates criticism and guilt, which is bad for your health.

Everyone does the best they can do with what they're given in the moment. This is a viewpoint that you can begin and end with. Wouldn't we all want and deserve the benefit of the doubt? We all want to do well, we want to succeed, and we all want love. If everybody's view was that we're all trying the best we can, then we don't ever have to challenge anybody's motivation. How can you complain about doing the best you can? That applies for everyone.

There are always circumstances that we don't understand that direct people to do the things they do. There are no random acts. We are directed one way or another by thousands of circumstances. It's just easier to accept that we can't possibly know the "whys" of life. So, instead of trying to make sense of something you can't, look at life through a filter of forgiveness. No judgment at all. Give everyone a pass for everything — absolutely all of it — at least try. It is a way to practice peace.

There's so many variables missing or unaccounted for. This is what makes us feel guilty when we judge — we just don't know. I try to remind myself that I know nothing for sure. When I say it out loud, it confirms the thought in me and my understanding of it. I am unclear about everything. I will try not to judge. I haven't seen, heard, or experienced what happened anywhere but in my own perception. I can't possibly know what happened to you. There's nothing that we can be sure of, except our freedom to choose what to think.

Be heroic in your attempts to forgive.

Boldly believe in goodness. Let all people shine — see only the best and assume greatness in everyone. We all are knowledgeable, caring, and full of kindness, but getting deep enough to see that isn't always easy. You don't have to. Just know it. Know in your heart that we're all one, all together, and all working towards our goal of being love itself.

There have been moments (although not very often) when I want to wallow in sad thoughts. I can't help myself even though I know it's not going to help me in any way. My viewpoint needs to be sad. At times like these, the thought of being happy pisses me off. I let it go. I get upset, and I watch myself be upset. I can observe and still be sad, but I'm never as out of control as I used to get. I know what I'm doing. I'm choosing sad thoughts, and I'm telling myself a sad story. I listen to my sad story, knowing I'm telling it. I don't believe it, but I listen. I know it's up to me to change the thoughts, and I do. Then it's over, and I'm back to being my positive self. That's all you do. You decide to choose different thoughts.

You are free to create your life with your point of view. This is our gift as humans. We can choose what we want to see and from which direction to see it. My point of view makes me who I am at this moment. If I'm feeling safe and loved, I am sending that out to everyone around me. It shows. My point of view is why you might want to be my friend, why I feel happiness, and why I'm healthy — it's physical and emotional. It's how I see my story, how I view the "facts" of my life, and how I respond. It's how I choose to view my world, and nobody can change it but me. It's only ever up to me.

I have a post-it note in my car. When I get in the car after a long day of work, the little note is sitting there, and it says, "Smile, relax, and use your imagination." I use my imagination to think of wonderful things, happy feelings, and healthy times. Where is the benefit to thinking an anxious thought? Really, let's examine why you would pick an anxious thought? It's all projection — no truth at all — imagination is all you're using.

I also have a sign in my house that says, "I am a figment of my imagination." You can imagine yourself to be anything you want. Shouldn't you use your imagination for better thoughts? Aren't you projecting anyway? So why not project positive thoughts instead of negative. We're just guessing. What possible good is it doing you to think negatively? Stop doing that! It's not good for your health. Anxiety comes from imagination. If you are right in the moment, you have no anxiety.

Loving life begins with gratitude, compassion, love, and forgiveness. If I change the viewpoint of myself, I can learn to override all those negative voices I've been hearing my whole life. *Why are you so gruff? So critical? Why can't you be more patient?* When I started finding compassion for myself, I could stop saying those things. I just stopped being critical of myself. I actually didn't even try; I changed from the outside in. I changed my behavior, and my inside voice stopped criticizing me. I had nothing to complain about.

– 39 –
Gratitude

Once I was diagnosed, I became aware of a gratitude that I had never experienced before — gratitude from just being able to open my eyes in the morning, gratitude to open a window and smell the air. Everything shines brighter when you aren't sure of your future. The opportunity to go see a movie becomes really exciting. I loved my kids, but not in the way I used to. It was almost like I could see them from a distance — they were just so wonderful as beings. My house, my garden, my work — my life, so dear and so precious. It became visible for the first time.

At one point, I was bald for the second time. The first six chemo treatments had not affected my tumors significantly, so I had another course of chemo scheduled, and I'd lost all the hair that was just starting to grow back. Then I lost all my eyelashes. It made me look pretty sick and vulnerable. I was thin and frail-looking. I was nowhere near done with what I was up against, but I was filled with a joy beyond anything I'd ever experienced. My body looked weak, but it wasn't — it was filled with joy and the purpose of living. My

213

heart was strong, my head was clear, and I was waking up looking forward to what the day would bring. The potential was almost unbearable; it was so wonderful.

It reminded me of when I was very young in the summer. I'd fall asleep with my head on the sill, listening to the cicadas, breathing in the outside air while my body was covered with just a sheet. I clearly remember the sand at the end of the bed from my dirty little feet. I'd lie there, cheek on the wood sill, waiting for the next day, so I could get out to the pond. I'd always be the first up in the house, waiting to begin the day. Excited for my opportunities — wondering how everyone else could be so blasé about sleeping through those early hours — I'd still have to wait for daybreak, and sometimes that seemed so long.

When I got a little older, I got tangled up in a confusion about myself, and, more importantly, what was dear to me. Even before all the doing of perfectionism, I lost my inner direction and became a follower of what was cool and proving I could be that. My friends didn't want to seize the day; they didn't find the pond inspiring. I stopped doing what made my heart sing. I forgot about my head on the sill. I couldn't find that sense of potential — I actually forgot it was there. It was all lost to me until I saw my life ending.

That thought of potential came back because of the cancer. My excitement to see the daybreak was there again. My fifty-year-old eyes would pop open in the dark just before dawn. I'd take blankets and go sit on the stairs of my deck and wait to be able to see the garden. I'd hear the crickets and the birds start. I'd breathe in the smell of the bay down the street and know that I'd found me again — that honest, innocent sense of Self that I felt as a child.

It was incredible to join with my old sense of Self again. Talk about an awakening! It has been so wonderful to meet up with me again. Of course, I was there all along, but I got lost in all the crap that I thought was important. It reminds me so much of my attitude now, feeling the looming potential of the day, the excitement of it. I am continually shocked at the possibilities available to me. I will not lose that fierceness ever again. I am fiercely alive now, and my sense of potential is going to stay.

There is a condition that has the opposite effects of post-traumatic stress disorder (PTSD). It's called traumatic growth syndrome (TGS), and it doesn't happen to everyone, but I was lucky. It showed me what I was missing. It cracked a hole in the hard shell of my doing, doing, doing, and showed me how to stop and SEE. Actually see people, events, and things for the first time in fifty years. It was truly an awakening. TGS is something that happens with trauma. This is the definition Wikipedia gives it: "TGS refers to positive psychological change experienced as a result of the struggle with highly challenging life circumstances." Some people, when faced with cancer or other highly stressful situations, have an extremely positive reaction to the experience.

I think that purposely working toward that kind of reaction is possible. When you have an illness, you have a choice just like with any other event in your life. You can choose to embrace it and learn from it, or you can wade through it just to return to your life as usual. Focusing on the positives, having gratitude, and finding joy where you previously saw misfortune can change how you act for the rest of your life.

By paying attention to the blessings in your life, finding gratitude in everything that comes your way, and believing in the goodness of people and all things, it's possible to turn cancer into a learning experience that is positive beyond compare.

The Optimists Creed
by Christian D. Larson

Promise yourself –
To be so strong that nothing can disturb your peace of mind.
To talk health, happiness and prosperity to every person you meet.

To make all your friends feel that there is something in them.
To look at the sunny side of everything and make your optimism come true.

To think only of the best, to work only for the best, and to expect only the best.
To be just as enthusiastic about the success of others as I am about my own.

To forget the mistakes of the past and press on to the greater achievements of the future.
To wear a cheerful expression at all times and give a smile to every living creature I meet.

To give so much time to improving myself that I have no time to criticize others.
To be too large for worry, too noble for anger, too strong for fear, and too happy to permit the presence of trouble.

To think well of myself and to proclaim this fact to the world, not in loud words, but in great deeds.
To live in the faith that the whole world is on my side, so long as I am true to the best that is in me.

– 40 –
Journaling

When I was diagnosed, it was a really busy time. A lot of change was happening quickly. I was concentrating on my body and my diet, and I was also learning what it was like to deal with breast cancer — the schedule of it. My life was filled up with appointments or getting ready for appointments. Every appointment felt like progress and was reassuring and somehow inspiring — another one down and less to go. Driving around to different places for tests and meeting with doctors took up many, many days.

During this time, someone gave me a journal. I knew that writing down all the doctor's appointments and dates was going to be necessary, but I also started writing down what I was eating and how I was feeling. This kept a log of what was going on with me on the inside and the outside. I began writing all the time once I was diagnosed. I wrote about everything physical in my medical journal, and then about everything else in my personal journal.

Keeping a journal regarding your appointments, treatments, surgeries, and comments made by nurses and doctors is a very good idea: what the doctors tell you, when the nurse explains something, how long you are told things will take — what you felt like during and after — all of your symptoms. These are all important to record.

The reasons are two-fold: first of all, at least in my case, there is a lot going on, and it can be a full-time job to keep track of it all. Hopefully, you are able to take time off or at least slow down your normal routine while you're in treatment. There are many things to remember, and healing takes time and energy, so a journal is a documentation of what you're doing that then enables you to let the details go.

Keeping appointments, taking medications, responses to medications and sleep patterns; foods that are working for you or not; your bodily functions and where you're having trouble — keep track of them all. You don't need to hold onto the factual side of this time in your head — write it down and let it go. Save room in your head for more important things, like spending time with your kids or friends, paying attention to your healing, and resting.

Second, it can be a kind of release to document all of it. The release is an emotional one and at a time where no amount of writing or journaling is too much. Getting everything down — how you're feeling physically and emotionally — is a way to promote your healing as well. Don't hold onto any feelings — write them, talk about them, and recognize them. Feeling them is important, but naming them is really important too. So writing about how you're doing every day can be cathartic and a great way to keep the facts straight.

People will be there for you, and they'll be a tremendous help and support, but no amount of caring people surrounding you can fill the space of fear. If you have fear, caregivers can distract you for a while, but it's still right there in your throat and only you are feeling it — it can feel isolating. It's a great release to be able to put that fear down on paper.

In the past, I had tried to journal but always gave up. I had tried buying beautiful notebooks, and then I'd try buying the perfect pen. I would write on the first page and hate my handwriting so much that I'd stop there. I tried buying spiral bound cheap notepads, and I'd use a pencil. I tried writing in script and in print. I bet I had twelve journals with one or two pages written in them. I was never able to write anything I could tolerate reading again, so I didn't ever continue.

I wrote with my left hand for six months. That way I couldn't be upset about my handwriting. The perfectionist never rests. I actually got pretty fast at it. Nothing ever satisfied me. I was embarrassed by what I wrote. Sometimes I'd open up a new journal in the middle and turn the book upside down — just to get started. That worked for a while.

I learned how to free write from Julia Cameron. Her book, *The Artist's Way,* which was written in 1992, and it's intended to be for people who want to develop their creativity. At the time, I was happy to do it, because it was about getting more creative, not writing, so it took some of the pressure off. Julia teaches what she calls "the morning pages." They are more of a releasing process than journaling. You wake up and free write, releasing what's on your mind. You ramble and babble if you want. It can be anything from what you have to do that day to a conversation you had, or that you have a sore throat. It's an exercise.

After clearing your mind, you leave room for creativity to come. This exercise, again and again, every morning, broke the journaling hang-ups I had, and I began to write every day. The morning pages were the beginning for me. Once I was able to write down all the unconnected things I was thinking, I broke through the wall. Julia says, "There is no wrong way to do morning pages." That was perfect.

Keeping a journal changed how I felt about myself so drastically in such a short period of time that you would have thought it was some radical new idea. Maybe that's why I tried so hard to do it for so long. At first, I was writing on plain copy paper, and I threw the pages out — big stacks of writing. I just threw them into the recycling. It was so much easier to know that I would never read them, and this was the exercise — you were supposed to just flush your brain of all the chatter. It was very freeing.

This kind of writing is very lose and unconstructed. You aren't going to read what you've written and that makes it easy to say anything. I started off that way, but it morphed into real journaling. That was cathartic, and I released anything I was too afraid to say aloud.

There were times when I could write about the cancer, but I couldn't have talked about it.

The journaling changed when I got cancer. It was part of the growth. It was obvious. It was me documenting the pain and the fear, and it became my emotional back up. The pages saved me. They helped me express what I might not have been able to. I remember I couldn't write the word "cancer" for the longest time. I had to allude to it, step around it, and imply it. Saying it and writing it made it seem bigger and badder.

Once I was able to write my feelings and daily musings — stream of consciousness with no sentence structure, I was able to let go of the self-criticism I had. I finally was able to write about what was going on in my life and not criticize my handwriting or how it sounded to my ears. I didn't care anymore, because it had changed me. That was about six months after I started the morning pages.

After about a year, I started using all the journals I had bought throughout the years, and when those got filled up, I'd write in anything I could find or buy. It doesn't matter what you write on. This is not "art." It's just your thoughts I always dated each entry, and this became very important to me later. When years go by, it's good to know what you were thinking and when you were thinking it. It's fascinating and uplifting to see your journey.

Keeping the appointment journal can literally be insurance against getting lost in the shuffle. The place I went to for treatments and surgeries had a fairly large group of physicians who all worked together. They would meet once a month to discuss each case and decide together what the right course of action would be. This kind of team approach made me happy, but I got lost in the pile of papers a few times. I realized that I had to be on top of my appointments and ask frequently how much time should pass between appointments and procedures. You need to be totally up to speed with your treatments and appointments. Although the medical community is supposed to be there for you, ultimately, it's your job to make sure the dates and places fit. There were a few times when I had to make a fuss about getting seen or getting a date moved for a surgery. The appointment journal really helped keep track of it all.

– 41 –
You Have You

Writing to yourself will change you. Keeping a diary, writing about your feelings or your emotions, creating a journal — whatever it is — a communication with yourself will change the way you feel about yourself forever. This is true — seriously, if you're honest with yourself on paper, writing will change your life. You will feel differently about your relationship with yourself within three months — I promise. It's life-altering.

In your journal, you can offer support to yourself. You can give the warmth and the love that you've always wanted from someone else. You say what needs to be said that only you know how to say. Know that you are the strength you need, and no one else has to fill those shoes. You know what to say to comfort yourself and ease your fears. Writing in your journal with brutal honesty will unlock your true nature and bring you back, so you can recognize yourself. You'll open up an avenue that helps you see your full potential.

Try writing it all down — all of it — document it. Write about the cancer, the appointments, doctors, your reactions, your kids, your relationships — whatever it is that's on your mind. It is an amazing time, and your thoughts are so revealing. Cancer is something to talk about even if you only talk to yourself — experience it fully and learn from it.

During the time I had cancer, I had me to talk to. I had me to turn to, and I did — every day. I was there for me. I had my back, and I felt a loving touch on my shoulder when I needed it. That's what writing did for me. Sometimes I could only say to myself what I needed to say, but it was enough to know I was there. In the loneliest and scariest of times, I could console myself and I knew what I was thinking. I brought something to write on everywhere I went. If I needed to express myself, I had a pen and paper, and I could connect with myself.

When I got diagnosed, the thought of getting on the phone with my closest friends, confiding in my doctor, my husband, my sisters, was too much at first. There was a truth that I had to tell that wasn't going to sound good — it was too dark and too emotional to share. I couldn't call anyone. I understood that it would be painful to articulate it — not just for me, but to whom I was talking to. There was nobody I could tell these thoughts to. I could write about it, though. I could think about it and feel it, and then get it out on paper. Just the act of writing it down is something good. I have thrown away many pages, because it was not something I ever wanted to read again, but I had expressed it and hopefully helped release it.

If you think you know what you're thinking, think again. You assume you know. You don't really know until you start writing it down. The fact of the matter is that you have an idea of who you think you are, and it's a picture — the story of you. You'll find out a lot you didn't know about yourself when you begin to write. The only way to prove this is to try it.

Thoughts are crazy — out of the blue, streaming in one minute and repeating for hours on end. Some thoughts are what you believe, and others are absurd. You already know you are not your thoughts. When you choose to write what you believe, you can learn amazing things about yourself. You are not what you think, but you are what you choose to accept. Big difference. You could go through a vast array of thoughts - hours and hours and believe none of it. What you accept as true is part of who you are at that moment. Change your mind and it's literally a different you.

When you start to write to yourself, if you're honest and lack self-consciousness, you will become your own best friend. This might sound too easy, but it happens. Everything you write becomes a way to share with yourself, and, as your understanding grows, your empathy and compassion will grow. As you write what's in your head and your heart, you will see you on the pages, and you will learn what makes you tick. Did you think you knew yourself? Maybe not as well as you thought.

You will laugh at your shallowness and your talent for complaining like a child. You will also be amazed at how much you think about things that mean nothing. Nothing! When you shine, you'll see it and smile. When you're brave, you'll be there to acknowledge it. The things that you do well will reaffirm your belief in yourself. When you're kind or misunderstood, it's you that'll know, and that becomes enough. It's the most wonderful discovery — discovering you. It's all documented — you're good, you're great, you're guilty, you're shameful — all of you right there on the page.

The best part about journaling is that it gives you your story. What is unfolding in your life? When you read it, you can decide what you think about that. Are you living the life you thought you would? Do you like what you're reading? You are completely responsible for the creation of your life, and you can alter and tweak it anytime you want.

– 42 –
Living outside the Lines

Nothing changed me faster than when I started to read my journal. I couldn't believe how much time I spent on things that didn't matter and never would. My morning meanderings were supposed to get thrown away, but when I stopped throwing them out and I'd read back a year, I realized that I still had a lot of growing up to do, and I thank those pages for showing me that.

I want to be a grown-up. I want to take responsibility for myself. I want to be someone I can look up to. I want to wake up excited with the opportunities I have today to be kind, gentle, and thankful. When I put my head down for the day, I want to know I've done my best. Journaling gave me that.

When I journal, nothing is off limits. If you edit yourself in your journal, you might as well be writing fiction. Honesty and truthfulness are key if you're going to learn from the writing. When it sounds bad or makes me cringe, I know its valuable stuff. Sometimes it was hard to read what I'd done, but then again, I knew that if I couldn't be honest, I'd have been writing for nothing. There is never any pressure to write something good.

Write what's real or forget it.

I wanted brutal honesty from myself. I didn't want to waste time being in denial, numbing and splitting off. I wanted to feel my feelings and move through them. I wanted to participate in my life on every level. I wanted to feel the uncomfortable feelings, and then be able to move past them — naturally and easily. I wanted to feel my anger, and then recover. Show me all of the hard stuff — this time I'll stay with myself, and I won't check out. I'll be there for me. I worked through all this with journaling and more journaling. I got me to face myself — it was so terrifying, but at the same time it was a beautiful coming home.

The biggest questions in my life come up again and again. Journaling about my spiritual beliefs are the ways that I grapple with my most frustrating and confusing feelings. It's a safe place to unwrap my complicated emotions, and resolution is not necessarily what I'm looking for. Praying, meditating, and journaling let me rest in my questions and ponder the "whys" of my life without fear. It's okay when there's no answer to my questions; I just have to go back to the same things again and again. It never gets tiring talking to yourself.

Anyone who considers this lifetime a journey would be smart to keep track of their travels. Your heart, your emotions, what you learn, and what you teach will be there for you to see. Reading your journal can remind you of what you've discovered and then forgotten. It's easier to remember how far you've come than to think of how far you have to go. Writing it down will help you see what you've accomplished. It's incredible, really, how much reading what you've done can give you confidence to do more. It's a fantastic book about yourself — really great reading!

When you write to yourself every day, you can see a bond building between you and your Inner Eye — your Self. I felt this happening, but didn't see it in my writing. I didn't need to see it on the page. It was pretty subtle, and it put a small smile on my face in the beginning. I can't explain the smile, except that I felt more like we than me.

When I read the writing that I did after the cancer treatments, I couldn't help but notice that it didn't sound like the old me. Of course, this didn't happen overnight. This is why it's so great to keep the journals. You can read and see where you've come from, remember certain times where you'd act totally different now, and see the lessons being played out. It's fabulous. When I read it, I could see clearly the shift in my character and mind-set.

Follow through was something that I'd had trouble with in the past, and through journaling, I owned up to that. I wanted to be there for myself as much as for others. If I said I would show up, I would because I didn't want to let myself down anymore. I'd be disappointed if I didn't follow through, and I didn't want to disappoint myself.

It never occurred to me to think about how I'd feel if I didn't follow through before. It never felt good letting myself down, but I never tried to analyze it. It's amazing that prior to that, I let myself down all the time. I guess I never considered that it was about self-love. That's what it comes down to, a respect and love for yourself. If you love and respect someone, you don't let them down and that includes yourself. And believe it or not, I got that through the journaling.

I was constantly talking to myself in my journal and rehashing feelings that I'd felt, conversations that I'd had. I started noticing patterns and behaviors that I didn't want anymore. I was becoming accountable for all that I did. It was easier to keep track of what I was doing when I was writing and reading about it. I was watching what I did, and then documenting it.

When I acted in ways that I liked writing about, I found that I would learn from that. When I did things that were hard to be honest about, it wasn't long before that behavior changed. If I couldn't change it, I would know I needed to work on it. It was amazing. I was happy to write it all down, because it was working magic. The shift in my actions was making me happier and feeling free of guilt.

Before cancer, I would have been unhappy to write my daily life down on paper. Being honest about my day would have been hard, because I was unhappy, self-centered, and driven by my ego. I wasn't living authentically, and, on some level, we all know if we're being true to ourselves or not. I was acting out a life that I thought I had wanted, but my heart was not there.

The journaling gave me a better sense of who I was, and I didn't like a lot of what I saw in myself or the picture of my life. As I changed my actions, I liked writing more and more. I enjoyed the time writing about all the things I was learning and what I was feeling. It was a kind of exploration of myself, and if I didn't like what was there, I'd work on it.

I think writing could be the single most helpful tool that I've ever come across to work through life's ups and downs. It has been a life-changer for me and unconditionally helpful — no matter where or when I've needed help. It's the journaling that's made it bearable.

Love after Love
by Derek Walcott

The time will come
When, with elation
You will greet yourself arriving
At your own door, in your own mirror
And each will smile at the other's welcome,
And say, sit here. Eat.
You will love again the stranger who was your self.
Give wine.
Give bread.
Give back your heart
To itself, to the stranger who has loved you
All your life, whom you ignored
For another, who knows you by heart.
Take down the love letters from the bookshelf.
The photographs, the desperate notes,
Peel your own image from the mirror.
Sit. Feast on your life.

– 43 –
Forgiveness

"Forgiveness is the means by which it comes to take the place of hell. In quietness it rises up to greet your open eyes, and fill your heart with deep tranquility as ancient truths, forever newly-born, arise in your awareness."

W-218 *A Course in Miracles*

When I decided to change how I was living, one of the first things that I did was make amends — just like in AA. Some of my memories were too old to fix and those I forgave in writing. The relationships I could do something about now were worth trying to fix in person.

If I could, I wrote or called people whom I'd had problems with. If I had a falling out with a friend, I called her and said I was sorry. I didn't defend myself — that was exactly the point — no story, just I'm sorry. I apologized and that was it. It didn't matter when or how the relationship had the problem. I was fixing it now.

Forgiving myself was necessary if I was going to lose my guilt and start fresh. Being forgiving of myself for my past behaviors was very difficult, because now I had a different idea of how I could have been, and it pained me to realize all my mistakes. I had done enough soul searching to figure out why I had been that way, so I could feel compassion for myself. Although I'd been controlling and perfectionistic, I knew I was doing my best, and I knew it came from years of fear. I forgave myself for everything I'd ever done. I really worked at it and wrote down everything I could remember. I wrote through it all, and every time I remembered another instance, I worked it through and I forgave myself.

Forgiveness comes more easily when you understand that there exists a grander scheme to the stories we're living. We don't know what part we're playing, because the whole script is unavailable to us. We don't know how we're affecting other players, and what the reasons are that things happen when they do.

We are not always here for the scene to play itself out — for it to make sense. It's so much easier to forgive and forget when you can just assume that there's more to what you see. Nobody hurts you on purpose even if it looks that way. There is so much more than you know. We may never know the "why" of a situation, and that's where your faith in people doing their best comes in.

Obviously, we've had things happen where people are not seemingly doing their best. People get hurt, sometimes worse. Life is ugly at times. People seem ugly at times. Those are even more reasons to be forgiving.

When I was nineteen, I was held up with a machete at my neck and a shotgun to my head. I was in Puerto Rico for Easter, and it had been raining for six days. My cousin and I jumped in the car in our bathing suits to go find the sun. We ended up in Guanica on Easter Sunday, four hours away from home. We got out of the car and started walking to the beach when three men came out of nowhere and circled us.

I had nothing but my bathing suit on, lots of jewelry, my 35mm camera, my purse with all my money, my plane ticket, keys for my car and my apartment back home and what you have in your purse on vacation — which amounts to everything worth anything. I was feeling very scared and vulnerable.

As they began telling my cousin (who spoke Spanish) what they wanted, I started to shake, and my legs gave way. I fell about four feet down off a little cliff onto the beach. They scrambled down to pick me up with gun and machete again at my neck and head. They picked me up, and I fell again, unable to hold myself up. So this was what "weak in the knees" meant. I had no idea it was a real thing. It was the opposite of scared stiff. I was so wobbly I couldn't stand.

They told my cousin they wanted the car, and my cousin pleaded with them not to take it. He told them we were too far away to be able to get home. He begged them to leave the car. They didn't.

They stole our car, took everything off me, except my bathing suit, and left us there at the beach. We walked over an hour to the police station. The police were clearly having an Easter celebration. I was very uncomfortable in just my suit; my purse, jewelry, camera and all were gone, but at least we were alive. It wasn't in the budget to get us back to my cousin's house. We had to wait for my aunt to come get us, and they hadn't yet answered the phone. The police didn't care much. They told my cousin that I would have probably been raped, but the muggers thought I had a physical problem not being able to stand up.

An hour later, the police asked us to get in the car, and they drove us to where the muggers had dropped the car off. They left the keys in the ignition. On the passenger side, a laminated picture of my dad that was in my purse had been left. I was struck with a feeling that they'd done what they thought was right. Isn't that funny? They took all my stuff and made me so scared I couldn't sleep for three months, and yet I felt they had done the best they could for their circumstance.

Now, here in my present situation, when I realized how important it was to forgive and continue to forgive, I saw how stuck I was on holding my story of being right. If you have trouble forgiving, try seeing if it's because you're sure you were right and they were wrong. This was my biggest forgiveness problem. I felt justified for holding people accountable for hurting me. All I have to do is remember; if you don't know the whole picture (which we don't), you'll never know what is right and what is wrong.

Holding onto old hurts is one of the best ways to create illness, and now I knew this to be true. Whether I thought I had justification or not didn't matter. I didn't want to make myself sick — I knew that holding onto old pain hurts the body. Right or wrong becomes irrelevant when you can't let go. Do you want to be right or do you want to be sick? If you have a choice to be healthy and detach from your grievances, wouldn't it be a worthy thing to work on?

Release all your burdens. Work on them. Forgive people. Write apologies to the people when you can and explain, but do not defend yourself — forgive and say you're sorry for whatever you can — for yourself – for your own sake. Forgive for yourself, but affect everyone by it. Releasing everyone from the responsibility of causing you pain is where your new life begins. It's not about them — it's about you, your pain, your health, your healing, and most of all it's your choice.

Nobody meant to hurt me — they weren't thinking of me; they were thinking of themselves. I knew this was true. Everyone is doing what they can to make it through their lives. Nobody sets out to screw up. We all do anyway. For every pain I had, I'm sure there was one I'd caused. I just had to remember that. There is nothing that can't be forgiven with time and intent.

Forgiveness is continuous. Forgiving doesn't happen once, and then you're done. Forgiving is daily, hourly — just holding it in your heart. Never not be forgiving — you're always forgiving. You should wake up ready to forgive yourself and everyone around you for anything. This is a practice. I have to work at it over and over again. I want to be open to forgive all the time.

I trust that by forgiving everyone for everything, I am going to hold onto my peace. I trust that by forgiving, I am also being allowing, and by allowing, I can accept everything. Allow as much to happen as you can and try to allow everyone to do what they want. Let things unfold and keep your expectations open. Keep your heart open.

Try to take everything a little easier. I remember the first time I heard the saying "rise above." I always thought it meant "be the bigger person." This creates an "I'm-going-to-forgive-you-because-I'm-the-better-person" feeling. I don't think so. I think it means "to use your higher Self to see the situation from a position that includes everyone's involvement." Rise up to a higher level, so you can see all parties as innocent and forgive yourself as well. When you rise above, you're literally seeing the situation with a bigger view so everyone is visible, and you can take more of the situation into consideration.

Trust completely with your eyes wide open and be ready to forgive everything all the time. At your most vulnerable, you are also the most free. I have a sign on my refrigerator: "Vulnerability is the doorway to God." When you feel wronged, relax. When you feel like someone hurt you, breathe deeply and relax. Can you feel your body stiffen when you feel hurt? Your heart tighten? You're holding yourself tightly, because you're in defense mode. Let it go. Take some time to feel the anger, hurt, and frustration, but then breathe deeply and feel it go. Explain to yourself that whatever happened did not go the way you think it did. Stop with the story of how it went down. Lose the story and you are free. You don't know what happened, and you may never.

"The secret of the ascent is to never look down
– always look up."
— Michael Singer "The Untethered Soul"

When you forgive, you offer your heart first. You love yourself enough to open to forgiveness because you know it's where you need to be. Love and forgiveness go hand in hand. You don't need to love the person you're forgiving. That's a plus, but it's not necessary.

Believe in love. We are all made of love. It's not a matter of learning how to love but a matter of relaxing our walls and resting in our true nature. Love is all of us, every part of us. We were made in love and we can't deny what we're made of. To find your loving nature, that was never gone, but gets built up around, you only have to relax into yourself. The love is there. You don't need to try, or will it to come. Open to it – feel your body relax and open to it, that's where love comes from – it's what you are.

When you get hurt, you close yourself off. Especially when you're very young, the hurt is more about physical pain and you learn how to close yourself down. When you're older and more mature and you realize that people are doing the best they can, you can understand better how to keep your heart open.

When you're truly open to love, the deepest connections are possible. When your heart is open, forgiving is done.

– 44 –
Lesson Earned

What happened to me when I came out on the other side of cancer was nothing short of a miracle. If you give up listening to your ego and just look for love everywhere you go, you will find peace and joy. Everything became easier for me once I knew how to find peace. I could replace my fear with love. My life took a different course.

I had been working on my life shift for about two years when I had a big fight with my daughter. I had changed since the cancer, but my daughter and I were stuck. She has always been the biggest teacher in my life whether I wanted it that way or not.

The fight included me telling her that if she couldn't be respectful and kind, she could move out. This came as a gigantic shock to her, and we were both out of sorts for several weeks over it. I knew I was wrong, because my heart ached, and I had learned enough to know this was a telling sign, but I didn't know how to fix it. I asked her if she wanted to go to therapy, and she agreed. I could tell she was anticipating major validation from the therapist.

After the first session, I knew that she would get what she wanted. The therapist was totally on my daughter's side to the point where I assumed the therapist had "mother" issues herself. My daughter explained to the therapist that her life had been incredibly hard, and a lot of it unfair, and I had made decisions without asking her for her opinion. She was really resentful and unhappy.

She said that I never listened to her, and I was always focused on my way of handling things when she had a problem. She said she had been miserable for years, and that she was depressed. Basically, everything that was happening to her was my fault.

I said that I had given her all I had to give, and her life had not been THAT hard. I said she was overreacting. I felt all my buttons being pushed at the same time — I forgot she was my biggest teacher — and I got swept into a defending position so fast it was too late to regroup. I started defending my myself and getting more and more furious..

The therapist got up and hugged my daughter with pity and protection. And while they stood there, arms around each other, she told me that I needed to listen to what my daughter was saying — clearly, my daughter had a point. I exploded saying that I had done the very best that I could possibly do, and how could that not be good enough? I then threw out some very bad language as I mentally started to shut down; I needed to retreat. I jumped up and left, which was my way of ending conversations that I was too afraid of or pissed off to continue, and it was something I had done many, many times in the past. The old behavior came back like I had learned nothing in the last two years.

I raced out, and several minutes later, my daughter came to the car. I knew at that point that I was wrong about all of it — the original reason for coming — and now the whole defensive, out-of-control reaction. I was feeling a lot of pain. I had acted so badly, and I had been so vehement — like another person had taken over my body.

In Eckart Tolle's book, *The Power of Now*, he calls this kind of reaction a pain body. Its painful memories stored in the body, and it will attach itself to the most current painful moment, bringing all the past pain with it. We all can identify with this pretty easily. It's when you overreact, and you can't figure out where all that emotion came from. It explains how you can act like a crazy person when you least expect it.

I knew the formula for peace. I had learned all this, but had seemed to forget it in a matter of minutes. I had to forgive and let go of why I thought all this was happening. I knew that I was experiencing the opposite of peace, and it isn't often we get to practice on the really big stuff. I was feeling SO defensive. I knew it was all about my ego trying to protect the "good mother" picture of myself. I knew it, and I still couldn't get passed it. My love for her had been replaced by my fear of not measuring up as a mother, being unlovable, and making poor choices for her. Which, looking at it now, were true to a certain extent, but facing it was so hard.

She got in the car. We had both been so upset, and we silently started home. I knew that if I got all the way home, we might never be able to fix this. This was not a little disagreement. This was a broken part of our mother-daughter relationship, and it wasn't going to get better without some serious attention.

The easy way to end it would have been to say I was sorry and try to put it past us, but it was so big and deep that I pulled the car over to the side of the road. I couldn't go home until we talked it out.

Shocking myself, I began by trying to defend myself again, like my mouth had a mind of its own. But then out of frustration, I started to cry. I told her that I didn't know how to be the way she wanted me to be. I couldn't see what it was that she needed. She was mad, but she saw my tears and my sincerity, and she began to tell me how she felt, and I listened. For the first time since I'd given birth to her, I really heard her. It was like someone finally turned up the volume on my deaf ears. I had never listened to her the way that I did at that moment.

I finally understood that by trying to help her by giving her advice, I had never heard her. I knew this scenario. I'd heard it before but I didn't think it applied to me. That was what she wanted though — validation. I was making her feel unloved, unimportant, and misunderstood by bringing up my experience instead of hearing hers. When I was giving her my advice, it was based on what I had gone through — all my stuff. Thinking my years of experience would help her, I would explain what I went through. But it wasn't about her — it was always about me — and she didn't care about my experience.

I listened to her talk about herself, and I didn't add anything. I wasn't trying to figure out what to tell her. I was just using my ears and my heart. I did it with love and compassion. And I felt compassion for me, too, because all this time, I had never understood what I was doing wrong. And now I did. I couldn't get it until I was ready to hear it. It was that simple.

It was as if I flipped a switch. With my defensiveness in check, I could really pay attention to hear her. When I let go of my ego's hold, I could choose to do the thing that would make me feel peace again. I wanted that feeling of having a light, unencumbered heart. I wasn't in this life to look good or to protect myself. Protecting is defending, and it's all about fear. I'm not scared of my ego. I'm not scared of what I'm doing wrong — I JUST want to do it right. I might be the biggest idiot on the planet, and the only thing worse than that is to defend my position.

Lesson earned!

I only wanted to love her, and I didn't need to get anything out of the relationship other than that. I didn't need it to be about me anymore. I saw that. I don't know if I had ever really seen her through neutral eyes before. I had always identified with her as "MY" daughter, not as a beautiful person without me attached at all. I took a lot of credit for her. My ego loved the way she validated me in so many ways.

I thought I was such a success until that therapy session. My mothering had turned out such a powerful, smart, beautiful daughter. I had a lot to be proud of here. But I was missing the whole point, because it had very little to do with me. I was only the vehicle that brought her here. Yes, I had helped raise her, but that had very little to do with now. I had put so much of my importance on her that I wasn't able to see her separate from me. There was such pride in me — my opinion and my history — it was impossible to let her express herself to me without me chiming in and adding what I thought was needed. Ouch! It was awful to see it.

When I looked at my daughter without me attached, she was just a beautiful person.

I can stop the story now. I can choose to just love her and give her my full attention. That's the best present I can give her. She's still my best teacher, but now I've grown to see where I missed before. I have learned to give to her, whether I get back or not, and to see her regardless of me. I still get tugged in the direction my ego wants me to go — but I have to say it's so much less. It's miraculous what happens when you see a story that perpetuates hurtful behavior, and you make a shift.

I want us to love each other, but not with anything attached to it. It is really only about me loving her, because if she didn't love me, I'd have to be okay with that, too. I can only work on me. I was finally able to see what had eluded me for twenty years — my daughter, as a person, just waiting to be heard by me, her mother.

"In my defenselessness my safety lies," says *A Course In Miracles*. When you feel the need to defend yourself, you're actually agreeing with what's being said. If you didn't agree, you could just laugh it off, but when you build up the energy to defend yourself, there is a part of you that feels there must be a valid point. Defending means you're not quite sure about your position and it's a great teacher. Learning how not to defend is extremely difficult. When you feel the desire to defend, that's the perfect time to see what's really going on. When your heart feels heavy, you know you've gone down the wrong path, and you can work on correcting it. There's no wrong way to get there; just opening up your heart for healing is sometimes enough.

– 45 –
Faith's the Opposite of Fear

Having cancer can be lonely because the people around you can't join you; they have to watch you go through it. Feeling lonely with illness can cause fear to come. Nobody can go with you even if they wanted to. No matter how supportive your family and friends are, there is no way for them to be on the gurney with you, lose their hair and eyelashes for you, or have a needle stuck in their arm for you. People can listen to you talk and hold your hand, but unless they've walked the walk, there's really no way for them to fully understand. It can be isolating and scary. The best way to battle the scary parts is to bring your focus to the moment you're in.

Although fear is about the future because you project what might be, it also has a way of making the moment stand still. Many things can bring you right to the present moment. Fear has a way of keeping you riveted to the here and now. I will never forget many of the moments I experienced during cancer. I can see them like they were happening right now. Cancer did that for me. Cancer gave me the experience of the present moment through fear — at least that's where it started.

There's nothing like fear to get you to pay attention.

When you are told that you have cancer, time stands still — you'll always remember those first few minutes. For most of us, I think it's surreal. Everything comes into focus like you've never known before. You can learn from that.

The present moment is a gift that once you cultivate a little taste of, it becomes something you look for. Allow yourself to slow down enough to notice where you are — smell the air, feel the sun, or see what's in your mind. Take a breath and feel your shoulders melt a little. It's an amazing shift. It's noticing a little part of your day or your life in an instant of time. I feel like cancer gave me the chance to see what the present moment was like over and over again. Just to rest there and be aware of it.

When I would get scared — right before surgery or even more often right when I woke up — I would think about the fact that nobody, not the most influential people on the planet, not the most spiritual people, nobody — has a guarantee that they'll live to the end of the day. None of us know our destiny. This I called the "great equalizer," and it always made me feel at one with everyone. It took the self-centeredness out of my fear. I didn't think of the fact that I had cancer and my chances of living through it were questionable. I considered my chances the same as everyone whether they were sick or not. It took me away from my self-focused thoughts and brought me out into a more expanded look on my life and the world. We are so

252

small and yet so great at the same time. We are all the same. It eased my fear.

"Don't give in to your fears," said the alchemist, in a strangely gentle voice, "If you do, you won't be able to talk to your heart."
— Paulo Coelho,
The Alchemist

I learned to notice my fear and remember that I don't know what will happen, so no amount of worry and imagination will help me figure that out. I am grateful for that. My path is not known to me. I have no idea what will be my last day, so I prefer to feel good right now, feel love right now, and be here right now. I breathe, I feel love, I breathe again. I relax into the moment. I don't think for a few seconds, and eventually I'm not afraid. Even on my scariest days of feeling alone and isolated with illness, I could find my way back pretty quickly by coming right to now.

Focus on what you can control. That's what will bring you contentment and alleviate fear. Whenever you're leaving the moment, fear has a tendency to see the opening and jump in. *How am I now? Right now? I could always handle the exact moment. Now, I'm okay. A minute later, I'm okay. I am sitting here, breathing and agitated, but I'm just sitting here breathing, and maybe a little less scared. I don't know what will happen in five minutes, but right now, I'm fine. I can handle it now…*and then I'd be okay. We all only have now. When you're scared of dying, now is a gift, because it keeps you from going into the future.

Fear is something we try to avoid. I'm not sure we should. What can fear do really? Fear doesn't have to be negative; you just need tools to deal with it. Gratitude has a vibration that dissolves negative, fearful thinking. You can soften the edge of fear by being grateful for right now. Coming to the moment that's here and not thinking about the "what-ifs" is how you can keep fear from eating at you. Being grateful for the moment you have right now puts fear in its place, because true fear can ONLY be about the future.

Don't be afraid of your fears. Fear doesn't need to scare you. You can observe and know that fear is only the misuse of your imagination. When you hold yourself in the present moment and breathe deeply, fear becomes a momentary uneasy feeling that just dissolves. Feel it coming and watch it, name it "oh, boy, that's fear I'm feeling." What's it doing to you? How does your belly feel? Is your throat tight? Do you have a crazy feeling in your chest? — lean into it and embrace it even, and let it just dissolve away. It doesn't last. It's trying to keep it away that keeps it coming back. Let yourself feel it and call it what it is. If you don't push it away, it's not as persistent. Feeling scared is okay — it's just a feeling. Feelings come and go.

"I must not fear. Fear is the mind-killer. Fear is the little-death that brings total obliteration. I will face my fear. I will permit it to pass over me and through me. And when it has gone past I

will turn the inner eye to see its path. Where the fear has gone there will be nothing. Only I will remain."
— Bene-Gesserit, litany against fear in Frank Herbert's *Dune* (Dune Chronicles, #1)

If your brain is looping a fear thought, concentrate on someone else. Make somebody feel good, give to someone, do a favor, and get away from thinking about yourself. Giving is how you receive. You'll feel much better and more centered when you've spent time doing things for other people. Dwelling on your fears will just create stress, and you don't want stress for your body. Remember that to heal you need to be in the growth cycle, not in the protection cycle. You want to feel grateful and relaxed to be in the growth cycle — that's exactly what you'll feel when you reach out to help someone.

When worry starts to trickle in, slow down and take a deep breath. Deep breathing will stimulate your parasympathetic nervous system (PNS), which will calm you. Remember that your body is completely connected to your mind. If you're in a fear cycle or a worry cycle, take a minute to really breathe consciously. Use this as a technique to deal with all your fear. Breathe. That's all it takes to move through your fear. It works. Stop fearing an outcome. Let all outcomes be possible — treat them all equally. They are only ideas in your mind. There is no reality in the future. There is only reality now. Breathe fully for a few minutes and feel your body relax.

In the book *The Healing Power of the Breath*, Dr. Brown and Dr. Gerbarg explain: "By voluntarily changing the rate, depth, and pattern of breathing, we can change the messages being sent from the body's respiratory system to the brain..." Messages from the respiratory system have rapid, powerful effects on major brain centers involved in thought, emotion, and behavior. You can change what you're dwelling on by breathing and focusing on your breath.

Having cancer gave me a lot of courage. Living through your fear gives you strength to be more courageous. When you live through a lot of "scary" things, you find you can face more than you thought. You figure fear out. Thoughts about death for months on end can give you a lot of courage. You get used to the idea, and then you get fearless. It was surprisingly freeing to feel like I had no control. I found myself doing things that I wouldn't have attempted before — showing up when I never would have had the guts. Being brave is so easy when you think you have limited time. It changes you.

You've probably heard that saying, "Do something that scares you every day." I like the thought of that, but it seemed a little daunting to me. I used to think that doing something that scared me meant that I had to go somewhere, start something, or perform somehow, but that's not true.

The greatest way to do something that scares you is to go into your everyday routine and do something different. Let go of control. Don't defend yourself. This is surprisingly freeing, but scary. Don't try to be right or better or smarter. Practice allowing someone else to be right, smarter than you, and more accomplished. Put your ego in the backseat for a little bit.

How about facing someone whom you know is mad at you and keeping your heart open. Running away was my go-to reaction for any kind of conflict. If I had an argument, I would stay away and make up all kinds of stories as to why I should. And I've faced that fear. I've overcome the fear of facing someone whom I've had a disagreement with and walked right over to them and said hello. I've sat next to someone when she was very mad at me and just sat there until a conversation started. Let me tell you, these are not little things for the woman I used to be! Nothing scares me much anymore. As a matter of fact, if I get scared, then I know I have to do it or face it.

The more resistance I feel, the more I need to go and do it.

The most important aspect about doing scary things is that they're usually opportunities for growth. What seems scary never plays out the way you thought it would. It is a way to push yourself to do things that you wouldn't normally. Get to know yourself better and see how you react. Take note of your stress levels and what is hardest for you. This becomes something you enjoy after a while. By watching yourself when you're scared, you take a big piece of the stress factor away. The act of observing, by itself, removes you a bit from the experience. Forcing yourself beyond the limits that you've determined for yourself is nothing but pure growth in action and scary! You can stay the way you are and march through your life thinking that this is you, the way you'll always be, and there is nothing wrong with that. But it is not "you." You are so much more than the body you wake up in every day. Your Self is constantly changing — your limits are in your head. There is a sameness to how you feel, so you think you're the same. It's all a game, really. You're only the "same" because you are physically feeling the same. Nothing is the same from day to day. There is no reason to stay the same other than its comfortable. A little fear never hurt you.

Don't be afraid of anything in the future, because nothing matters more than what you do right now. Nothing about the future is important right now. That will be what you're doing then, and you'll be busy. There's a saying, "Worry is a misuse of imagination." Remember that and think about it when your head is full of the future and what might happen. All fear is future-base and you're not there now.

The fear of having to leave my life woke me up. There is no such thing as a typical experience for someone diagnosed with cancer. We all find our own way. I was very driven to recover this is true. My diet, the research, and all the books on spiritual growth had infused my life with a newness that gave me hope and purpose. My feeling of responsibility gave the experience a twist I had not expected. I had watched my parents and grandfather die from the disease, but I never saw the change in them that I realized was possible until I saw my own.

– 46 –
Sharing Your Truth

Being humble is not about hiding your gifts or downplaying your achievements. It has nothing to do with making yourself smaller. Not a thing. Being humble means being honest about everything — your weaknesses as well as your greatness. No one is just great. Nobody does amazing things without doing stupid things as well. Hiding the things that make us all human is what limits our relationships.

What you don't share about yourself is as important as what you do. Hiding parts of yourself — editing who you are — is just as though you were pretending to be someone else. When you don't show who you are, all of who you are — your weaknesses, your shadow side — you keep a wall up to others around you. If you let the wall down and admit what it is your trying to protect, you give everyone else permission to do the same, and that's when you're real. You cannot expect anyone to be real around you when you're protected.

Be accepting enough of people so their truth is always able to show. When you feel accepted enough to be honest, you can develop a deep relationship. Being vulnerable and honest opens up the same energy for everyone you're with. Hiding from your vulnerability just keeps everyone else hiding, too. There is no way to honestly share if you don't admit who you really are. Being critical of yourself will keep people from sharing. You think that you're just criticizing yourself, not them, but they see you judging yourself, and it keeps them from sharing with you.

"The privilege of a lifetime is being who you are."
— Joseph Campbell

I never showed my vulnerable side to anyone. Somewhere in there, between all the doing and busyness, I shut down. Looking back on it, I can see a couple of reasons, but they're not important. The important thing is that I thought it was safer for me to stay tough. I couldn't get hurt if I was tough — this is what I thought, but it was also not true.

The truth is that it's just as easy to get hurt when you're tough, but you miss out on all the good stuff when you're hiding your sweet side. Staying tough keeps everyone at a distance. When you keep trying to be a superstar and trying to be better, you never end up connecting with other people, because you're so busy trying to prove yourself — you separate yourself. The only way to join is to be vulnerable and soft to situations. My friend Sharon always says, "soften, Kim, soften".

When the only side that you show is your strong side, it keeps your relationships on a surface level. That's not the whole truth. There may be less pain, but it is lonely! Where there's no depth, there's no sharing either. You can't be only part of yourself. In order to have a whole relationship, you have to be all of yourself.

I used to beg my husband to talk to me. He couldn't tell me what he was thinking, because he never felt me share the way I was asking him to — it would have been too hard for him to show weakness when I was only being strong. All he saw was me always in control, disciplined, and holding it together. He couldn't talk to me nor would he have wanted to. I needed to be vulnerable in order for him to open up, and I wasn't.

When you share your weakness and your shadow side, bad behavior, and mistakes, you give everyone else an opportunity to be honest about themselves. No one feels free to share their blunders with someone who appears to be doing everything well all the time. When you don't share everything, it takes away all the honesty from the sharing. To have a full, deep relationship, you can't omit things, because the parts you leave out complete the puzzle of you. Leaving holes in the picture leaves you incomplete, and it's obvious. It creates space where you want closeness. People will always sense whether you're giving the full picture or not.

I made so many mistakes hiding my weaknesses. Being a perfectionist will do that to you. It'll take all the fun out of your screw ups. I hid my difficulties, my compulsions, and my true feelings. From the outside looking in, I looked pretty good. But that was the problem. If I'm hiding my weakness, I appear really strong, and that appearance is a lie. You can't connect with lies.

When I would show just the pieces of myself that were doing well, I shut out everyone who wanted to be real with me. My perfectionism was keeping me from being honest with myself and with all those around me. What is the point of any relationship if you don't have honesty? Really — what's the point? You don't know who you're dealing with. If you don't know them, then it's all just a game. There's no moral code — no integrity.

"Perfectionism is not a quest for the best. It is a pursuit of the worst in ourselves, the part that tells us that nothing we do will be good enough — that we should try again."

— Oprah

By hiding your mistakes, you take away the opportunity to balance your relationships. Who wants to admit a fault to someone who is "always right"? We all fail, we all fall down, and we all have parts of us we'd rather not admit to. This is a beautiful part of our humanity — it's the balance — admitting our faults and having a sense of humor about it, then moving on. Doing that makes it easier for everyone to be humble and honest, and then really share in your glories, too.

If you hold yourself to a standard that is practically impossible to maintain, it'll make it hard to admit to yourself when you fall short. You won't have a lot of relationships who'd share their not-so-perfect life either. It's no fun when being honest about yourself means you're the only one in the relationship talking about failing or not measuring up.

When you are humble, you are not dimming your brightness, but merely admitting when you weren't shining.

Sharing the parts of you that shine is only welcomed when you've been honest about the other parts, too. Being honest about what you learn in your self-searching is what helps our relationships to grow stronger. Staying humble and honest about your shortcomings is the best way to develop intimacy in all your relationships. Not shying away from the parts of you that you find uncomfortable takes bravery. Being honest takes courage. Knowing your true self and owning it, really staying with it, is where your power is. It's right here, in this moment of utter honesty.

The closer you come to knowing yourself, the less fearful you become. Knowing who you are inside and deep down will bring you a sense of wholeness you never dreamed you would have. Staying in the same painful place sometimes feels unbearable, but that's when you have the opportunity to know yourself — by not avoiding you. Sitting with yourself when you're uncomfortable and not running away is the first step towards self-love. Being honest and welcoming of all of you – your beautiful faults along with your glorious virtues is what makes you whole. When you recognize the love you have for yourself, you can be honest about your imperfections. Not only is it easy to admit to your shortcomings, it's part of what you love about yourself.

– 47 –
Authenticity

When your soul starts to stir, and it wants to be heard, there's not much you're going to be able to do to stop it.

It's not like a whim; it's more of a demand. It steps from the background of your consciousness into the foreground of your life, and you can't ignore it. Your interests shift — your thirst for purpose comes into focus, and yes, you change. You can't help it. Some of us change to such a degree that our lives can't continue on the way they were going. Your career might end, your marriage may break, or you may move 2,800 miles away (or even all three).

When huge change happens, everyone who knows you wonders what's up. What is she doing? And you think the same…Who am I? Am I really doing this? When big things change like your body, your marriage, your business, your home, and who you are, you feel uncertain. If everything else is changing, how much am I changing too?

I was very late coming to this party — the soul-stirring one. I got diagnosed with cancer two months after my fiftieth birthday. I may never have realized how consumed with the minutia of my life I was if it weren't for a serious, face-slapping wake-up call. I began to change before I even found out for sure that I had cancer — the mere mention of it had me in motion.

I started to perk up when conversations shifted to things of a spiritual nature. New books, courses to take, and new ways of seeing things all had my attention. I read more, attended meetings, and found people who felt the same way — which happens naturally when you're energy shifts. Situations appeared, books literally fell into my lap, and my energy began to attract a different sort of person.

The people in my life changed. My twenty-five-year marriage ended. Although my life was still about "me," it was now about my purpose, and it felt deep and full of meaning. The feeling of needing purpose didn't go away and still hasn't. I am open to new things, new people, and most of all new ideas about how my life is unfolding, what it means, and what it's going to look like. I have changed beyond what I thought possible. My personality is, at times, unrecognizable from before — so what?

Your life is here now just waiting for you to take the trip, to make the commitment, take the leap, and make it a joyous thing. The joy is not at the end — it's in the process, the planning, the doing, and yes, the commitment! Don't wait for time, money, or permission. You own your place here on Mother Earth — you own it.

You are all that matters to you; it's hard to fathom that. But when you come into your own life, your own head, and your own path, you are actually helping all those around you to do the same. I'm not talking about being selfish here; I'm talking about being authentic.

With love in your heart and an open mind, you are the be-all and end-all of your life. Get rid of your guilt, your resentments, sadness, and most of all your victimhood. Take charge of what you want, who you are, and where you want to go. Don't wait for the end of your life to come and hear yourself say, "Oh, I could've..."

The goal of your life is not to reach a goal.

The goal is to make your experiences while you're living the best, most present, heartfelt experiences possible. The goal is not at the end when you've achieved something. It's not up ahead in front of you. The goal is in each moment — right here — right where you are. Striving towards a goal gives our lives excitement and purpose, but it's the underlying experience — the everyday experience that will matter in the end. Your goals are secondary. It's your way of life, the WAY you spend your days that makes your life an expression of your true self.

In order to create an amazing life, you have to want it and know that you can get it — one day at a time, or better yet an hour at a time. You make your life amazing with your thoughts. It's less about what you do and more about how you feel about what you do. Small steps turn into big things. Decide that you want an incredible life. You can have whatever you want. Think of the potential!.

Don't strive to be something outside of yourself. Strive to be yourself — the best you can be without changing who you are. Strive to honor who you really are, and then see where that takes you. You were born to be you. Trust that you are perfect beyond and underneath your story. The story is what is giving you the trouble. Make decisions based on who you love and what you love, and then follow your heart — leave your history out of it. Don't be afraid. Don't hesitate. Don't judge your life. Life will not wait, but there is no rush. There is no better time than now. You won't be ready later, tomorrow, next month. What can you do now to start doing what you want to do in this life? How can you share your wisdom and your gifts? Even if it's just changing your attitude about what you already have, do it.

> "Do not let your fire go out, spark by irreplaceable spark, in the hopeless swamps of the approximate, the not-quite, the not-yet, the not-at-all. Do not let the hero in your soul perish, in lonely frustration for the life you deserved, but have never been able to reach. Check your road and the nature of your battle. The world you desire can be won, it exists, it is real, it is possible, it is yours."
>
> — Ayn Rand

– 48 –
Creating Your World

Bringing creativity into your life starts with noticing that everything you do is creating. Be open and accepting, curious, observant, and discerning. Notice and decide on what appeals to you. Trust your unique ability to notice what only you can see and appreciate. Trust that everything about you is just as it should be. Only you can see your wisdom and then speak your wisdom. Get to know it, and then begin to share it.

> "It is not the end of the physical body that should worry us. Rather, our concern must be to live while we're alive — to release our inner selves from the spiritual death that comes forth living behind a façade designed to conform to external definitions of who and what we are."
> — Elisabeth Kubler-Ross

As you decide on your likes and dislikes, understand more of who you are — who you were born to be — your confidence in your "taste" will build. The more you get to know yourself, the more your taste will be your own. Your likes are your own — don't judge them. The ego is what judges. Start to recognize this and shut it down — it defeats the whole purpose of finding yourself. Comparisons are of the ego, and the ego knows nothing of your true knowing.

As you create, you evolve. As each of us creates, we all benefit from the creative action. The world moves forward with every act of pure creation. The more expressive we are, the more in touch with our inner consciousness we'll be and the more the world in general evolves.

You grow through creativity. The importance of being an individual is most obvious when you consider growth through evolution. Our world needs to grow in order to move forward. Humanity needs to grow to evolve. Mainstream living and conformity does nothing for growth. We need to grow through our uniqueness. It's the only way. Your ego will try to curb your creative ideas to keep them "safe," but that's the opposite of what we need. Your authentic self is what is needed in the world right now. Nothing created with ego will be authentic or dynamic. The ego squashes originality. Self-centeredness is not a place you can create from. Bravery and courage in your own ability, uniqueness, and originality will enable you to truly create.

Being open and free with new ideas gives everyone around you permission to do the same. Think of it as a creative purpose — to help others grow through their creativity. We should be helping everyone to be themselves. When you begin to show your creative side, it opens up the world for your friends and family. This sharing helps everyone create and helps the world evolve.

Your house and your surroundings — your car, your yard, and office are extensions of you. They have energy. Your house protects you; it reflects you. It takes on the energy of you and your family. Things take on your energy when you use them, wear them, and live around them. They can nurture you and restore you, or they can drain you and sap you of your precious time and energy. When they are expressions of you, they'll nurture you. When they are inauthentic, they'll sap your energy.

Making your house reflect the energy you'd like is not hard if you lose the fear of being different. Surround yourself with colors that make you feel good. If you have favorite clothes, notice their colors. Using colors that are in fashion is conforming and not authentic. Painting a room with a color that you love reflects your energy. Think about what you want to do in your house — where to sit, do projects, read, or relax. Once you decide what you want and need, you can arrange your house to reflect you. What do you like to do, and where would you like to do it? We have houses that have entire rooms devoted to things we do once a year. How crazy is that?

When I got cancer, I moved all my sewing things to the dining room, and I never moved them back. Didn't it make more sense to have a sewing room if I did it all the time? Also, I had a very nice living room, but I couldn't stretch out or dance. I took the furniture out of the middle of the room, so I could stretch out, dance, and meditate on the floor. I was able to use the room all the time for what I did every day. I loved being able to really move in my house. Honestly, who is living in the house, and what do these people do? Take the time to make the spaces work for you and fill your life with good energy.

Cabinets, cupboards, drawers, your desk, the garage — all these places are parts of your life that can drain you. You have the ability to make them areas that uplift you and be tremendously helpful. Drawers can be stressful. Everything drawers — the drawers with all the junk from everywhere — takes up space in your head. Do you have three or four of each utensil in your kitchen? How hard is it to find your favorite pan? Do you have to sift through a lot of stuff to get what you need? You need to edit. Give things away, donate, and clear your space or extra things.

Seriously, these things drag on us. They actually deter creativity. Too much stuff drags you down and changes your flow. You open a drawer to find a paperclip, but there's everything and anything — papers, five pairs of scissors, or no scissors, because they're all over the house in strange places. Nothing makes sense. It takes away your energy.

Clear out the drawers and get rid of stuff — it'll clear your head and help you make room for bigger things. It's healthier. It'll make you feel lighter and more open to possibilities. Getting rid of clutter releases all kinds of stress. It's healthy. Picture the difference between opening a drawer with five pairs of matched socks versus twenty pairs that are old, no good, not matched, and not worn. Stress is not healthy. You know which socks you wear — get rid of the rest.

Don't cling to what you don't need.

Do not underestimate how much stress is lifted with organized and pared down living spaces. Too much in your house creates too much in your head. There's no place for peace. When your living and working areas are more spacious, so is your head and your heart. There's room to be spacious. There's room for peace. Peace is healthy.

Every time you make changes to simplify, more peace will come. The material things are only the beginning. When you make changes to bring more peace into your life, your body will respond and appreciate it. You can say that you are actively creating peace in your life every time you give things away, donate what you don't need, clear out a drawer, or have only what you really need. You are using your energies to create the life that will bring you peace, and then joy and creativity. It is incredibly uplifting to let go of feelings and of possessions.

It's not all about giving away. Choose what you want to keep with care. What matters to you is important, and what doesn't should go. If you keep less around you, make it beautiful and meaningful. Nothing lasts forever. It's just stuff. If you knew that it didn't matter, none of it, then you could let it go.

Cancer puts all these things that you "have" in perspective. What will all that stuff do for you in the end? Isn't it more important to put your focus on what's living and breathing? Your beautiful house should nurture and comfort you, but only to a certain extent.

When it becomes stuff that you're clinging to because it feeds your ego, you need to be honest about that. Am I just impressed by what I've picked out? I'm good at decorating, right? Don't I do a darn good job making my house look pretty? Does this really mean anything? To whom? Think about it. You're impressing people for what? When's it going to count? Does someone tally up all your good taste at the end? Worry less about how it looks, and think more about how it feels.

I know I was caught in that trap. I was proud of myself for doing a good job. I was living through the image that I was projecting with my house and my possessions. There is nothing wrong with having a beautiful house, but when those things define you — when you are so identified with them that you can't imagine being who you are without them, then you've got a problem. They're just things, and when you're gone, it won't matter what you've picked out or how much stuff you had. It doesn't matter how long you live; you don't get to take it with you.

When I thought I might die, I never even considered my stuff. I thought about my kids, my sisters, my family and friends, my dog. People. Things that breathe. That was it. Not what I'd leave behind — not things that I made or bought, kept, or inherited — none of it. Not what I'd accomplished, painted or written. It just doesn't matter. What matters are your relationships.

The word "inspire" means to be in spirit. Your house and your clothes, your food, garden, job — whatever you do that you put your mark on are all potentially inspired by you. When you can make decisions based on your likes and what inspires you, you show your own authentic true self. This matters and makes your life have meaning. Put your mark on your house and your style, but don't define yourself with what you have. It's fun; it's creative and that's it. It's something you can do with love and care but not connected so much to your ego. There's a difference. You're motive will let you know where you're coming from. Have fun with the looks of your clothes, your house, your garden, but don't take yourself too seriously — it's just stuff!

Are you trying to prove yourself or are you expressing your true nature? Think of yourself just as yourself — with none of your things. You're whole and perfect without them, and you must always remember that things don't make you who you are. Spending time proving yourself is a waste of time, but expressing yourself is an excellent way to be creative.

Your true self is what needs to be met with acceptance. If we all worked at showing what makes our hearts sing, we would be much less apt to ridicule anyone. Once you've made the effort to show your individuality, you'll never judge anyone who's doing the same. You know what it takes to show yourself and the strength it takes to go against your ego. Admiration will flow through you instead of criticism.

Expressing yourself takes guts and courage. When someone judges you in any way at all, it is because of fear — fear of being judged. Its okay — don't judge them for judging you. Really, they don't know — allow them their opinion. If you continue on, it will open up a new view for the people who judge. They will learn from you. Judgment is never about the person being judged, it's always about the person doing the judging. Once you see this for the truth, somebody else's opinion means almost nothing. The only opinion that matters is your own.

– 49 –
No Such Thing

Never limit your ambition to what you know how to do. There are no limits at any level of your experience, except those that you choose to make. When you listen to your ego, you are creating limits that don't exist.

It's fear of the unknown that stops you in your tracks, or maybe fear of success and fear of failure as well. There is nothing to fear. The other side of success is failure, but if you never try, you'll never achieve either. The actual "trying" is what living is all about. If we challenged ourselves, and "went for it" all the time, nobody would worry about failing, because we'd all fail and move on. It's the people who spend their lives trying that are really living.

"I do believe that we know our reason to be here. We don't know if we are taking the exact right steps toward it. But if you are honest enough, God will guide you." Paulo Coelho who wrote The Alchemist during an interview with Oprah

Have you ever tested your limits? You can push yourself to the edge, but when you get there, are you done? Is there really a limit? How would we know? We don't usually go there. We don't do the things that scare us, because we're afraid of failing. The other side of "fail" is "succeed." You can't get to "yes" unless "no" is a possibility as well. Who cares why you think you have limits — all you have to know is that you don't know until they're tested. Our limits are in our heads. What you believe will be what happens. If you feel limited, you are. If you feel limitless — go towards that — have no boundaries.

Are you so committed to your image that you are afraid to grow?

We need to look for and find the authentic you under all the busyness — all the obligations and the false yous. We have a lot of roles to fill: wife, mother, friend, daughter, sister, boss, worker, partner, creator, athlete, cheerleader, and so many more. These roles do not necessarily resonate with the original you. They limit you. By definition, roles are limits. They are such a part of our lives that we forget about the first "you" that defined who we were. That little kid who couldn't wait to get out of bed in the morning is still in there somewhere.

When did we lose track of our individuality? Somewhere along the way, we forgot who to pay attention to. We forgot where we were going, and we veered off in another direction, away from ourselves.

We forgot and we kept marching along, proving our worth and performing, and then all of a sudden this person was there who couldn't remember who we used to be. What do we do? We continue on, blindly going to work, raising kids, blindly following the way everyone else is going — living out our lives — and missing that original spark that we used to have — our uniqueness that no one else on the planet has but us.

I held onto that. I held onto the fact that what I was doing looked a lot like what other people were doing — so it must be right. Right? I conformed because I didn't know any better. I followed what my parents had done, and sometimes exactly the opposite of what my parents had done — which made it seem even better — but it wasn't original. The life I was leading wasn't different; it was pretty much the same as everyone else, and for a while it was okay.

My authentic-ness started getting lost in the shuffle somewhere between getting out of college and getting married. If I could have stepped back and taken stock in where my wants and needs were at that time, I might have been able to reroute, but I don't think I could have been honest with myself at that time. The limits that I had put on my life were familiar in that I recognized them in everyone else I knew. I was doing what I thought I was supposed to do. I was totally okay with no originality, it seemed to be working fine.

Being the only person ever in the Universe to have your genetic makeup, your history, your Karma, and your belief system puts you in the perfect position to be only you. Like Oprah says, "I've got Oprah down."

Nobody else can be who you are. You are perfect at being you. Finding out what you really want to do, who you want to be, and how you want to act doesn't have to happen at any specific time — there isn't a time frame. Some of us aren't ready until much later in life. Some of us just start with originality and never lose sight of it. Some of us need to get sick to start showing up. It's never too late to figure it out. You can really work at it or just dip your toe in and wear a different hairstyle. This isn't about right or wrong. This is about opening up to your limitlessness.

Open yourself up to new things and learn where you have hidden desires, tastes, and potential. Learn new stuff — read about things you know nothing about and see where it leads you. There are no RULES. Do not be run by routine. Branch out. The things that are unique to you should be shared, and the more you know about your uniqueness, the better. Sharing who you are on a genuine level is what gets you back to that authentic person — who you were born to be.

A lot of us have been fitting in and playing roles for so long that we don't even know what we like. We don't feel limited, but we act that way, as though the rules are given and we blindly follow them. I think this has a lot to do with limiting our decisions to those that will be okay with everyone else. So few people are willing to stick their necks out and be true to themselves. I know it because I've done it, and it comes at a cost.

Maybe you won't fit in if you decide to follow your own music. Maybe people will criticize you, or maybe you'll end up finding the people you have the most in common with, because you didn't hide your beautiful colors. Put yourself out there — see what blows your hair back. Make deep footprints and stop caring about who's watching. Be pleased with yourself. Don't be timid. Risk it — it's worth it.

The Universe isn't interested in you acting out a life like you're in a performance of how grown-up and enlightened you can be. The real, true you with all your inadequacies and blunders — that's the YOU that needs to show up and face your life. There is only one you, and there'll never be another way to express yourself exactly this way. This is it for right now — you in this particular body at this particular time. Down the road, is anyone going to care about how you rocked your own boat? Will you be remembered for your fearlessness? For your color choices? For the fabulous gardening you did? The classes, travel, acting? Where does your authenticness show up in your life? What's in it for you?

We unconsciously believe that the right way to live is what everyone else is doing. If it's outside of the norm, it somehow is socially wrong. We basically let everyone else tell us how to live. We mold our lives to conform, and we're conforming to what? Someone else's idea of what's right or normal? Where's the trust in our own minds? Nature made us special, God made us special so shouldn't we embrace what makes us different? We bend so we don't stand out at all — but whose opinion matters more than our own? Who's living this life — who is it that matters more than you? Do what you want to do now or get to the end of this spectacular life and wish you had? Does that make sense?

Getting sick can be an indicator you're not fulfilling your authentic calling. You're off balance. And when you get sick, you get the courage to find it — those things that make you exactly you. After I was diagnosed, I became a driven woman. There's no fooling around now. Threaten my life and I'll start to wake up every morning with an agenda. My life might end? Seriously, NOW you have my attention. What was I waiting for? Do we have to wait for chemo to be all we can be? What can I do to make my life more authentic? Because if I don't have all the time in the world, I'm going to make it count right now.

"Why fit in when you were born to stand out?"
— Dr. Seuss

We are here to discover our true selves. We are born to push the boundaries of what we think we can do. We are here to prove there are no limits. We are here to make a contribution. We are here to embrace connection with the other people like us, to share what we are and what we learn. If you're busy fitting in, you are not doing that. What is the point of being you if you aren't embracing what makes you different? It doesn't make sense. When you hold back from being who you truly are, who are you really living for? And the best question is: do the people you're living for really care about how well you fit in?

"To be nobody but yourself in a world which is doing its best, night and day, to make you everybody else means to fight the hardest battle which any human being can fight; and never stop fighting."

— E. E. Cummings

– 50 –
Finding Your Tribe

When you get to the place where you love yourself more than you worry about opinions, you can make decisions based on what makes you different, not what looks like everyone else. When the love for yourself comes, so does the need to be seen as who you really are without fear and without shame — no excuses or defenses. When you become comfortable with the idea of your being unique and perfect just as you are, you're drive to be seen as only you can be seen will increase.

You'll naturally become more individual. You'll naturally stand out more, but you'll be happy about it. People will start to ask you where you bought your clothes and compliment you on random things. Did you change your hair? You didn't but you're radiating a unique energy now. You'll get noticed and that's the point. Your friends and family will see the real you in your house, what you wear and your style, and in time your courage will give them the permission to express themselves, too. This is SO important.

We are here to help each other to be ourselves. This isn't a one-man show — you do it to give the people around you the courage to do the same. We all need to shine. We all have the ability to be perfectly different, and we have a responsibility to share ourselves so we'll all grow.

Conforming is an act of self-denial. It's denying your Self. To conform, you must deny your true expression. When you really love yourself, and you let your true nature come through, the act of conforming is less appealing. Why shouldn't I be original? I love who I am, and I want to express that. You can only get over your self-consciousness when you love what you are. You can only really live the life that you should be living when you can let go of everyone else and their opinions.

I'm very fond of the idea that the Universe doesn't support hiding. It will back you up every time, but you have to give it your all. Show your stuff. Make a big statement. Shine your light. Don't be scared to say, "This is me!" Tell it like it is.

The more authentic you are, the more you connect with people you are meant to connect with. Expressing yourself is the opposite of hiding. After cancer, the fear of getting out there was dramatically less with me. Whatever! Who cares? What's more important than being myself? Think about the reasons why you don't go for it. There isn't ANY reason that makes sense. Be who you are born to be.

You are constantly creating. There is never a moment when you aren't creating your life. When you put on your clothes, your makeup, your jewelry, when you make the bed, wash the dishes, make breakfast, make the coffee, creating is what we do. But we lose sight of our freedom with it. You are choosing thousands of things a day that make your life just yours. Do you realize that? When you move, you create. Everything you do is creation at work. Make those choices be your choices, not choices so you're like everyone else. You are different and you can't help it, so own it.

So many of us go to the extreme to fit in. We eat the same foods, go to the same stores, watch the same shows, and act the same way. We pretend we like things, because they're what our friends like. We get stuck in a rut and go along with everyone else, because it takes more energy to be an individual. What better way to use your energy.

Conformity is a way to feel safe.

It's safe to hang out in a pack. It's safe not to stand out in a crowd — to blend in. If you don't stand out, you're probably less likely to get noticed, and the ego likes that. The ego will talk you out of wearing something because you haven't seen it on someone else. It's scary to be out of the pack until you look at the reasons why you think that. It's hard to stand out until you embrace why you are the way you are. Why else would we be made this way? We were made to stand out otherwise, we'd all be born the same.

– 51 –
Risk It

L iving without risk is like saying you're healthy because you aren't sick. Health is not the absence of disease in the same sense that feeling fully alive is impossible without some kind of risk. Never taking a risk will suck the life out of living. Risk puts the contrast into life that you need to point to what is possible — good or bad, alive or dead. It's the contrast that makes us feel vital.

Nothing makes you feel more alive than jumping off the cliff of an idea and being responsible for the outcome. Serious risk tests our abilities and reactions, making living through the experience one of growth, anticipation and excitement. You risk something, and then see it through, and you have surpassed a possible limit. It's life-changing every time, and it builds your courage.

If you don't take risks, you'll never be able to see what you are capable of. Learning about your capacities — mental, physical, and emotional — is the most exciting part of being alive. To not take risks is to deny the reason why we're here on this planet — to grow, to learn, and to experience what life has to offer in order to find out where, if at all, our limits are.

Install new beliefs into your daily mental talk. "I can absolutely do this." Lean into the difficulty and be happy about it. Learn to push through your resistance and risk it — whatever that means to you. Do you want to start a business? Can you risk learning a new language? Can you cook something with an ethnic flare for thirty people? Submit a piece of art to a show? Enter a contest? Here's your shot to be original and inspirational.

"Whatever you can do or dream you can, begin it. Boldness has genius, power, and magic in it."
— Goethe

Why strive to be something outside of yourself when what you find inside is what you were born to be? Instead of trying to be someone else, strive to honor who you really are and see where that takes you. Be true to your inner nature and get used to listening to what really makes your heart sing. I realize now that standing out is what draws the people you need into your life. I need those people in order to be a better me.

We connect with our energy. You need to be seen exactly as you are in order to meet people energetically. If you don't show your true nature, you're just connecting randomly with people — nice, friendly people, but not the people who will empower you to be more of who you were meant to be. When your energy is true, it's a whole new ball game. It's not about who you like, but more about who resonates with you.

Standing out is how we attract the people who will resonate with us. You can't attract the people into your lives who will help you grow unless you show your true colors. Doesn't this make sense? Your tribe are the people who think like you. They are the people who will make you feel like you're the coolest person around. They will support you and help you nurture your uniqueness. You cannot find your tribe unless you put yourself out there.

To stand up for what you love and show it is where you build the inner you. You can develop a love for your uniqueness — so much so that standing out becomes something you strive to do. Iris Apfel, a fashion icon, is an idol of mine, and she totally understands the magnitude of being true to yourself. I apply what she says to everything in my life, not just what I wear. What do we have to lose? Live to please yourself and no one else.

"I say, dress to please yourself. Listen to your inner muse and take a chance. Wear something that says, 'Here I am!' today."

We have to do our best to listen to our hearts and create what we're driven to create. We have to be authentic with our inner calling and respond to where we need nurturing. We have to move beyond just caring for everyone around us and create a life that reflects who we really are and what we really want. This doesn't mean we neglect our jobs and the people we care for. It just means that now they really see us while we're doing that. Owning your point of view takes risk and courage, but it gives all who see you do it the permission to do the same.

Self-expression and being authentic are rightfully ours. The more unique you are, the more inspiring you can be. The balance that we lack after years of taking care of a family and being a partner is usually in the area of expressing our authentic selves. I was being creative every day, but I had lost my true sense of self. I was playing a role and didn't know that even though I created that role myself, it wasn't me — it was who I thought I should be.

> "There is a force within you that gives you life — seek that. In your body, there lies a priceless jewel — seek that. Oh, wandering one, if you are in search of the greatest treasure, don't look outside. Look within, and seek that."
>
> — Rumi

A good way to see if something is authentic is if it takes no effort. You love doing it so much that it takes nothing to do it. When something is completely easy — no effort required, no strain to get there — it's probably authentic. I don't mean lying-on-the-couch-watching-TV easy, I mean trying to find those things that feed you — your soul, who you're meant to be. When you lose track of time doing something — that's what I'm talking about. Losing track of time while you're busy is the true definition of happiness.

"All things are possible to those with faith and courage. As I believe in my heart so it shall be done unto me." This is a quote that I've tattooed around my right forearm. Believing in my heart is why I monitor my thoughts — I make sure I'm thinking from the heart and not the head. If I have faith and courage, and I believe it, nothing can hold me back. I watch my thoughts and make sure they mirror what I believe. Have faith and courage — that is the answer to all your questions. Don't squash your dreams, don't underestimate, don't limit, and don't listen to the thoughts of your ego.

– 52 –
You Have to Remember You

There comes a time when you begin to realize that you've been paying so much attention to so many other things beside you that you're not really there. It looks like you're right there, but really the essential you is missing. You're immersed in the doing. You're so focused on what has to get done that you've become an afterthought. We all get stuck — it's the yin to the yang. In the beginning of our lives, we know who we are, and we're totally focused on ourselves. Then we go so far to the other side that we have to regroup, back up, and turn around.

I seem to remember somewhere in my twenties, when I was still enjoying the outdoors, that I was still going boating, camping, and thinking of how I would spend my time off. I can vividly remember planning time to sit in the sun. At that time, it was a worthy plan. That didn't happen once I had a family.

At some point, the time off became a reason to get more done. I'm assuming marriage had something to do with it — as if now I had a serious life and I better prove it. I know for a fact that once I had two kids in fourteen months, I was busy for the next sixteen years doing things. Life took over, and instead of me planning it, a lot of it planned me. I know I let it happen. I had choices, but I made the choices based on how it all looked. I definitely did things because they looked good.

Much of my life seemed to be the culmination of a bunch of errands, working, and a clean house. As I got older, I kept wondering, *Is this it? Where's the good stuff? How did I get here?* When you're busy all the time with your family, job, and household, the doing can just take over. I missed a lot of important moments. I was very busy playing my role. I'd forgotten how to be that original me and sit with the moment. I'd forgotten the one who had time and plans to sit in the sun. Doing can be a valuable thing, but that busy kind of doing doesn't have a lot of value. It's a distraction to avoid connecting.

When and how this happened is a mystery to me. I know that my sense of worth was tied to it. The doing was a way to prove myself. Everything I did made me look more deserving of love and admiration. My kids looked great, my husband, the house, garden, my work — it all added up to a more substantial me. Right? You could just look around and get an idea that I was doing just fine, maybe better than fine. The problem was that I wasn't really doing it for me. I was doing what looked good.

At my breaking point, I had been on a role that had lasted for twenty years. I don't know why I didn't realize that I hadn't been there for myself. It wasn't anyone else's fault. I orchestrated the whole thing — completely ensconced in the "life" I thought I wanted. Did I just change my mind or lose my mind? The question is irrelevant when you're breaking. Once you realize that you've lost what's inherent to "you," you panic trying to get it back and wonder if it's even possible.

Getting cancer was the impetus for finding me again. It forced my breaking point. What a gift! When you're faced with the possibility of your end, the whole of your life comes into focus. You do an overview. You kind of say, "So, how well did I do?" What's important, what you've done, who you've loved — the good as well as the crummy. Looking back, I found I was happy with a lot of my past. I had done my best, but even doing your best can leave out what's important. Not too many complaints, but I couldn't really put a finger on what seemed to be off-kilter — something was missing. And then I realized it was me.

Finding yourself can be the best thing that comes out of this whole event. I realized with a shock that I was alone, and if I was so sick I might be leaving this life, it was going to be by myself. Does that sound crazy? I just never faced it before. It was a real eye-opener, and it was what started the whole shift of seeing my inner self.

If it was just me, then I better start paying attention to what I came here for.

If it was just me, then everyone else was doing it for themselves, too. I had to be true to myself or die trying. I found myself alone with myself, and it all started to click. When you're super busy, you don't get the benefit of being alone with yourself. If you don't give yourself the time to feel alone, you'll never face yourself. It was me sitting there with me, and I finally liked it.

I negotiated through a lot of darkness by listening to my inner Self. I will never again lose that part of me. If I can't find a place where I feel real and well, I'll make one. I won't settle for only a part of what I want ever again. There's no reason not to have the life I want. Most of us don't know who we really are, because we're so busy trying to conform and stay inside the lines that we miss the opportunities to shine. Living outside the lines is where the real living is — where you can express your true nature.

Being worthy of love started with me. I had to love myself first. If I couldn't love myself, how could I expect anyone to love me? That's crazy. If I don't love myself, I can't even know how to really love someone else. Show yourself love. When you give love freely and stay vulnerable, the love will come back to you. If you want love, don't look for it. Give it. You get what you give. If you give it, it will come to you.

My mother didn't understand self-love, and I learned from her. She understood that the only time you were lovable was when someone loved you. If she wasn't getting love from someone, she was unlovable. That is exactly what I grew up thinking. Someone else determined if I was lovable or not, but not me. Being able to love yourself by yourself is the beginning of love itself. There is no other way to get to real love. It doesn't take another person to have love — it comes from within you. It is always there; you just have to tap it. You don't create it; you look within.

Being true to your nature brings what is meant to be yours to your life. When you release the outcome and let go of control, what is meant to be yours comes to you, because you've opened up enough to let it in. Forcing your ideas on how things ought to be delays what you're meant to have and do. Being exactly as you are and letting events flow creates the energy that enables things you need for your authentic Self to come into your life. When you try to force situations, you create a false energy that doesn't match up to who you are and where you are meant to go.

> "You develop an enthusiasm for no longer watering those negative seeds, from now until the day you die. And, you begin to think of your life as offering endless opportunities to start to do things differently."
> — Pema Chodron

– 53 –
Grounded

February 2, 2013, was when I saw the whole life I'd been making fall apart. When the details of our financial disaster had been worked out to the best of my ability, I left my house and moved in with my aunt and uncle on Cape Cod. I put all my things in storage. I took a few clothes, a little furniture, and my border collie and drove away. I asked them if I could stay with them for six months and they said yes. They were very kind to share their beautiful little house with me. It was April when I landed there.

I decided that I needed to work outdoors and get my hands in the dirt. I knew this didn't make a lot of sense to most. One of my sisters said, "Oh, I'm so proud of you." I couldn't figure out what she meant. A fifty-three-year-old woman working on a landscaping truck is hardly something that would raise a feeling of pride, but I guess that was all she could think to say.

Working with a gardening crew seemed to be exactly what I needed, and it surprised me to think of it. I wanted to get physically powerful and work so hard that I couldn't think forward or backward because both of those directions presented huge obstacles for me. I had been a pretty serious gardener my whole adult life, and I felt sure this would be the best way for me to heal and escape at the same time.

I started working for a small high end company in Chatham, Massachusetts, on April 17. The company maintained some of the most beautiful gardens on Cape Cod. When I was hired, there was concern that I wouldn't be able to handle the physical strain of the job. I had twenty years on my boss and thirty-plus years on the guys working in the crew. I had a two-week trial period. It was the second coldest spring on record for the Cape. It didn't snow, but it came close. I kid you not — it rained every day for the first two weeks of work.

During those first two weeks, we never saw the sun. I had two coats that I wore at the same time, two pairs of gloves, two pairs of socks, rain pants, a hat, and a neck warmer. I learned for the first time in my life that you could work all day soaking wet. We worked really hard for eight to ten hours with half hour for lunch. If you took a break, it was to sneak off to pee in the bushes. Many of the properties were on the ocean, and, of course, the gardens were amazing. Some of the properties were so extensive that our crew worked there twice a week for hours on end.

My job at first was the same as everyone else's: hauling huge barrels to the truck, raking, pulling weeds, and pruning. I never knew how hard it was to dump a garbage bin full of wet yard waste into a dump truck until I had done it for the twentieth time in one day. I learned there's an art to it and to icing sore muscles.

On the first day of my second week, I was asked to rake the sand underneath a deck so that it looked neat from a distance. It was so windy that day that the rain was pelting me sideways. I had to lie down on the ground, in the mud, and extend the metal rake as far as I could under the deck, pulling back and forth to level the wet sand. Talk about initiation. I was sore for at least a week. Every night, I'd put bags of frozen peas on my elbows and wrists to get the swelling down.

I made it past my trial period and went straight into spring planting and pruning, which meant hours of digging in the mud and cutting back hundreds of hydrangeas. During May and June, we worked ten to twelve hours a day. I wore a uniform and brought a back pack with my three favorite pairs of gloves, bug spray, sun block, an extra hat, full rain gear, lunch, and two forty-ounce stainless steel water bottles. I was given a leather holster for my Felcos, and before long, I looked like I had been on the job for years. I was brown from the sun, very strong, and so sore at night I couldn't do anything but frozen-pea my muscles and crash. As I walked in the door every night, my aunt would say, *"Do you have to pea?"*

By the end of June, I was driving the truck, working on my own some days, and very close with the whole crew. My boss had stopped testing me and would use me as a "fine-tuner." The whole process of getting up in the dark, getting to the jobs, knowing what I had to do, tending the gardens, loving the land and seascape, coming home, icing, scrubbing to get rid of ticks, and falling into bed was deeply satisfying. For the first time in my life, I ate like I deserved it.

While I was working for the landscaping crew, I was also learning Italian. I had so much new information coming in that it was thrilling. I couldn't wait to listen to my tapes to and from the job. And then, while at work, I continued to learn about the business of landscaping.

It made me think a lot about how we get to be a certain age and we're really knowledgeable. We are all smart in what we've concentrated on. We put our focus on things, and that's what we learn. But at a certain point, a lot of us stop learning. Is it because it takes effort to learn new things that we stop? Or because we only want to look smart? Is it because we usually don't get paid to learn?

We can keep adding to that reservoir of knowledge. I didn't want to keep doing what I'd been doing for the past thirty-five years. I wanted a change. Until you focus on new things, you forget what it's like to have to really pay attention — to memorize and remember what you've learned, to be tested, to be the new guy.

I realized that I'd stopped learning anything major. Being a beginner can be a little daunting, so we tend to avoid what we don't know about. My ego loved knowing so much about what I'd been doing, but it wasn't too keen on being a beginner. It came to me that learning a new job, learning a language, and living somewhere new was not hard — it was just adjusting to the new input. We forget that there's no end to what we can learn. There's no end to our capacity to take in new information. Learning was exhilarating.

The last day of my job on the Cape was on September fourteenth. I had promised my boss five months, and although it was a hard summer, I will forever feel thrilled that I worked that job. My dream of being a "bad ass" was fulfilled when my boss said she'd keep me on if I wanted to stay. She wrote me a recommendation that brought tears to my eyes; it was so beautiful and heartfelt. It made me realize that I could do anything I wanted to.

I had decided to go west. It was only in the last few weeks of August that I really made up my mind. My legal issues were not over but they had settled to where I could move, the divorce was final, and my time at the Cape was coming to a close. I flew out to Arizona on the seventeenth and rented a little house. I looked for a job, but I knew that it might take a while. I spent a week hiking and getting to know the area better. I loved it so much I was sorry to have to go back and get my things.

When I got back, I packed up my car and drove across the country with my girlfriend, Lisa and my dog. The moving truck with my possessions came a week later on the eleventh of October. I moved in and looked around. All the things that I had learned in the last four years were in play now. I was fearlessly starting a new life 2,700 miles away from "home." I didn't know anyone, but I didn't need to. I had me and that was enough. I felt full of goodness and promise. I joined some groups, signed up at the library, got my license, and registered to vote. I changed my mailing address and started my new life.

"The most important thing is to hold on, hold out, for your creative life, for your solitude, for your time to be and do, for your very life; hold on, for the promise from the wild nature is this: after winter, spring always comes."

— Clarissa Pinkola Estes

– 54 –
A Different Level

W hen I got cancer, I had all the energy in motion for my life to unravel. There was nothing to do but let it all unfold. If things were going to be different with me, then everything that happened had to be dealt with on a different level. What did happen was all part of the fallout from those years of resentment and a misguided mind. I'm not saying that it was all my fault. I know that it took a whole lot of bad decisions to get us into that place, but I will take responsibility for my part in it. I had to accept that what was happening to me I had brought on myself.

My ex-husband probably tells another story, and his lessons are his to tell. I believe we were brought together to learn what we needed to learn and to give life to two amazing kids. We had twenty-six years together, and many were very good. There is no anger or resentment for me that I can tell. I have forgiven all of us as much as I can for this moment. Tomorrow, I'll have another chance to forgive again. My experiences put me in the right place for many events to be seen clearly, and if I didn't learn the lessons yet, then they'll come back again and again until I do. I think he was my soul mate.

"A soul mate is probably the most important person you'll ever meet because they tear down your walls and smack you awake."
— Elizabeth Gilbert

Into each day, I bring what has hurt me, inspired me, taught me, and tortured me. Where else could I be but here? The real question is: would I want to be anywhere else? What sense would that make? Who am I to argue with what I need or how much I can stand? Trust in the process of life to bring you right to the center of where you need to be to find what needs to be found — to learn what might be learned. My girlfriend Maggie says that true personal change is like an iceberg. It's so slow that you can't tell its moving, and most of it is beneath the surface. All I'm aiming for now is to be awake enough to move through my life gently with love and honesty — whatever else happens is beside the point.

How I choose to view my days is where the beauty of possibility comes in — the unbelievable potential sitting right in from of me. What a gift — this life. Being given a breast cancer diagnosis can be nothing short of terrifying — but it doesn't have to be. Life is iffy. You don't know if you'll wake up tomorrow. You take what you can get. You enjoy when you can and see the beauty all around. Your days of good health are embraced, and the days you suffer are spent one moment to the next. It is naively looking at your life, with innocence and wonder that brings joy. Look at everything as a miracle. Take nothing for granted. See with fresh eyes every morning. Pray for peace every night.

After I made it through the whole ordeal, living my life seemed a breeze — a gift, really — and gratitude filled me up and made me smile. People kept saying it would go away, the feeling of gratitude. But when it's acquired, it'll stay if you want it. You don't have to have cancer to be grateful.

Most of all, the journey that cancer took me on made me wonder where and who I was before. How much I had missed avoiding the moment. What was I doing with my life? Cancer gave me the courage to be more vulnerable and unknowing, so I could really look at my life with wonder. Being vulnerable was the scariest thing for me before cancer. I know now that I won't vanish if I get hurt. I won't disappear into pain if I fall short. I know that if I get knocked down, I'll eventually get back up — and probably with a smile on my face. I'll still be here to feel it and get through it. I'm as invincible as I'll ever be. Vulnerability is where I'm open enough to experience the true nature of relationship with all its connection and possible pain — the real deal. I want that. I'm not scared of anyone anymore.

I hear little echoes in my head of regrets, but they're few. I can choose to rise above them. I forgave myself for everything, because I understood all the reasons I had to do what I did. I spent years wasting time being self-consumed when I could have spread more goodness. But in the end, I just wasn't ready to be different than I was. We are all doing the best we can do — ALL of us. If you can stop and just think about that; that we're all on a path of understanding and growth, no matter what it looks like.

Let your guard down enough to express who you are. You are not alone. You have gifts that need to be seen and shared. You are unique and now you can be fearless. Now you have even more reason to share your stories, your creations, and your abilities. Be bold and be brave. Show your stuff — show your uniqueness. Live in the moment, because now you know that's all we have. Find your voice and find your style. Express yourself. Show others who you truly are and inspire others to do the same. Tell everyone what you know.

My body said, "Hey, I tried to tell you, then I tried to show you, and now I'm going to make you finally see what you need to see." There is no question that being diagnosed was the first step in the greatest journey of my life. I wouldn't trade my experience with anyone…just like you would never trade your kids — they're yours. My cancer adventure was exactly what I needed, and I loved it. And, yes, I said that. I loved it. It changed me forever. It brought me to God, to goodness, to positive viewpoints, to forgiveness, and mostly to love.

> "You cannot change your fate. You can, though, rise to meet it."
>
> — Lady Eboshi,
> *Princess Mononoke*

Made in the USA
Middletown, DE
09 July 2015